AUSTRALIAN MARITIME SAFI

MW00749073

# M/V „RIG SEISMIC"

# Survival at Sea

# A TRAINING AND INSTRUCTION MANUAL

An AGPS Press publication

Australian Government Publishing Service
Canberra

© Commonwealth of Australia 1993
ISBN 0 644 24262 0

First published for Department of Transport 1978
Reprinted 1979, 1980
Reprinted for Department of Transport and Construction 1982
Reprinted for Department of Transport 1984
Second edition published for Department of Transport and Communications 1989
Third edition published for Australian Maritime Safety Authority 1993

National Library of Australia Cataloguing-in-Publication data:


Survival at sea.

3rd ed.
Includes index.
ISBN 0 644 24262 0.

1. Survival after airplane accidents, shipwrecks, etc.
I. Australian Maritime Safety Authority.

613.69




Printed for AGPS Press by Dix Print Pty Ltd

# FOREWORD

Australia has always relied heavily on the sea for commerce and communication. Although the sea has a friendly aspect, it also has a merciless side and is unforgiving of the carelessness, neglect or incompetence of those who sail on it. Safety at sea must be the constant aim of all seafarers, and knowledge of the effective use of life-saving appliances on a ship is a major step in achieving that aim.

In 1978, the Commonwealth Department of Transport published an instruction book to help prevent loss of life at sea. This book, *Survival at Sea: Instruction Manual*, was well received and has been reprinted several times.

Since the original publication substantial amendments have been made to international safety requirements. These and other changes have been incorporated into this new edition.

*Survival at Sea* is intended to be a useful and effective aid aboard ship and ashore in training seafarers in the use of shipboard life-saving appliances. Whilst primarily intended for those aboard trading vessels, much of the information will be of use to persons on fishing vessels or recreational craft. It is a handy reference to many techniques relevant to survival at sea.

Paul McGrath
Chief Executive
Australian Maritime Safety Authority
Canberra

# INTRODUCTION

This manual describes the various types of life-saving appliances carried on Australian ships, their operation and the general survival procedures to follow when abandoning a ship at sea.

This knowledge is of vital importance to every crew member on every ship. Every crew member is therefore given a copy of the manual and the chance to learn by reading, discussion and practice how to survive and to help fellow shipmates survive.

Knowledge gained from this survival manual is to be supplemented by all crew members attending at survival courses, musters and drills, which will further educate them in the safe and expeditious use of abandon ship procedures for the various types of survival craft.

The type, number and location of life-saving appliances on Australian ships vary considerably according to the type of ship, operational area, size and age of ship, manoeuvrability and the number of people carried. Federal, State and Territory marine authorities take account of such factors when exempting ships from carrying certain appliances and when allowing them to carry appliances considered equivalent to those normally laid down in Marine Orders, State or Territory legislation.

As a result of the changes to SOLAS 74 consequent on the 1983 Amendments coming into force on 1 July 1986 there are generally three different standards for life-saving appliances on Australian ships. These are for (a) new ships, i.e. those of which the keel was laid on or after 1 July 1986, (b) older ships, i.e. those where the keel was laid earlier, both (a) and (b) being under Commonwealth survey, and (c) intrastate vessels, fishing vessels and pleasure craft, which are under State or Territory survey, and where the standard is generally in accordance with the Uniform Shipping Laws Code.

In addition, the introduction of the Global Maritime Distress and Safety System (GMDSS) in February 1992 has caused a difference in communication equipment standards between non-GMDSS and GMDSS fitted ships.

The manual is generally aligned with the standard for new ships, but refers also to the standard for older ships. Most material is applicable to all ships. It is important that each person is fully aware of the number, type and location of the life-saving appliances available, and is familiar with the various alarm signals which may be sounded in case of an emergency. In addition, each person should ensure that the lifejackets carried on the ship can be donned correctly.

## Acknowledgements

The Australian Maritime Safety Authority (AMSA) gratefully acknowledges the assistance of the maritime industry in preparing the second edition of *Survival at Sea: A Training and Safety Manual*, and comments provided during the preparation of this third edition.

The Authority also wishes to thank shipowners for permission to use photographs of life-saving gear aboard various ships, and manufacturers for permission to reproduce illustrations and drawings from technical literature. Where possible these are appropriately acknowledged in the manual.

Finally, AMSA acknowledges the kind assistance provided by the St John's Ambulance Service in updating the first aid section of this manual.

# CONTENTS

# List of illustrations

# Chapter 1

# Stowage of life-saving appliances, organisation and training

This chapter covers the stowage of life-saving appliances and the training and organisation of personnel for an emergency situation. When a ship is at sea all life-saving equipment must be kept ready for use at all times. It must be maintained and tested or inspected to ensure that it is in working order. Ship's personnel should report any defects observed in life-saving appliances to a responsible officer.

## CONTENTS OF THIS CHAPTER

## STOWAGE OF LIFE-SAVING APPLIANCES

### Lifejackets

A lifejacket is stowed in each person's accommodation. Additional lifejackets are stowed in working spaces such as the engine room, bridge and forecastle and in float-free lockers stowed adjacent to the lifeboat and liferaft muster stations.

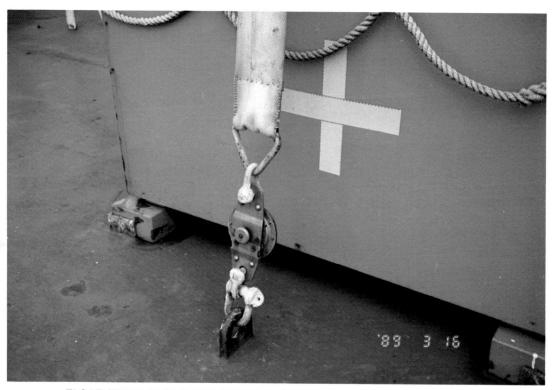

FLOAT-FREE LIFEJACKET LOCKER SHOWING THE HYDROSTATIC RELEASE
Courtesy: BHP Shipping

Each lifejacket is fitted with a whistle, retro-reflective tape and a light powered by a water-activated battery. Each person is required to know how to put on a lifejacket correctly and how to operate the light.

## Lifebuoys

Lifebuoys are stowed so they can be quickly  thrown overboard in an emergency. At least half the lifebuoys on a ship have self-igniting lights attached and there is at least one on each side with a buoyant line not less than 27.5 metres in length. These lines should not be lashed with twine or rope yarn, but kept free for immediate use. Most ships have a lifebuoy in a sloping rack on each wing of the navigation bridge. These lifebuoys are for use when a person falls overboard at sea. When a securing pin is pulled out the lifebuoy, which is equipped with a light and a smoke signal, drops into the sea.

## Immersion suits

An immersion suit is a protective suit which helps reduce the loss of body heat of a person wearing it in cold water and is designed to prevent the wearer from receiving a shock on entering cold water. The suit covers the wearer's entire body with the exception of the face and is meant to be worn over normal clothing. If the immersion suit is made of material which has no inherent insulation it should be worn over warm clothing.

Some immersion suits have inherent buoyancy or inflatable buoyancy chambers and are designed as lifejackets as well as immersion suits; others have no buoyancy and must be worn in conjunction with a lifejacket.

Immersion suits have generally been required since 1 July 1991, though not on ships with totally enclosed lifeboats or ships constantly engaged on voyages in warm climates. However, ships built, or fitted with a rescue boat, since 1 July 1986 require an immersion suit for each person in the rescue boat crew.

Ill-fitting suits and difficult inflation devices can cause problems. All crew members should be instructed in the use of suits carried aboard the ship.

## Thermal protective aids

A thermal protective aid is a bag or suit made of waterproof material with low thermal conductance. It is simpler and, in most cases, far cheaper than an immersion suit. It covers the whole body of a person wearing a lifejacket, except the face.

The wearer should be capable of removing the thermal protective aid within two minutes while in the water.

Carriage requirements for thermal protective aids are generally similar to those for immersion suits.

## Buoyant apparatus (existing passenger ships only)

Buoyant apparatus is distributed about the ship in positions where it can be easily launched overside, or can float free.

## Liferafts

Both inflatable and rigid liferafts may be carried on Australian ships. There are two types of inflatable liferaft: one is thrown overboard, then inflated and boarded in the water; the other is inflated at deck level and lowered fully loaded by a special davit.

Most liferafts have a strap or lashing over them to secure them in their stowage position. If fitted, this strap or lashing must incorporate either a hydrostatic release or an equivalent automatic release system. The exception is the additional liferaft carried as far forward or aft as practicable and reasonable on some cargo ships, which need only have a manual release.

A hydrostatic release is a device activated by water pressure which releases the securing strap at a depth of about three metres. If a ship sinks with a liferaft in its stowed position the release opens and allows the liferaft to rise to the surface. Hydrostatic releases must be fitted with a means for manual release, such as a lever, push button or pedal, or a separate slip.

Some hydrostatic releases, such as the 'RAFTGO', are spring loaded and require to be correctly tensioned in order to ensure that the release will operate. Those responsible for rafts (and float-free lifejacket boxes where these are fitted with hydrostatic releases) should ensure that when rafts are restowed after servicing these releases are correctly tensioned, and that the tension is correctly maintained during the voyage.

Non-davit-launched inflatable liferafts have fibreglass outer containers. These are usually carried in cradles or chocks at the required stowage positions although they may be placed in racks or chutes. The stowage is designed to make it unnecessary to lift the liferaft when launching it. A simple means of levering the liferaft out of a cradle and over the side may be provided. On small ships where the deck on which the liferafts are stowed does not extend out to the ship's side, a ramp or guide to take the liferaft over the side is provided

# INSTRUCTIONS

1. Take suit out of bag and open fully.

2. Don as normal coverall.

3. Kneel to fasten leg zips.

4. Fasten waterproof zip fully to neck.

5. Don hood and fasten face cover.

6. To vent suit, turn valve anti-clockwise and press down.

7. To vent all air, adopt crouching position.

8. Suit is always to be used with an approved lifejacket.

9. Remove gloves from arm pouch.

10. Don gloves and zip up.

The suit is now fully donned and ready for immersion in water.

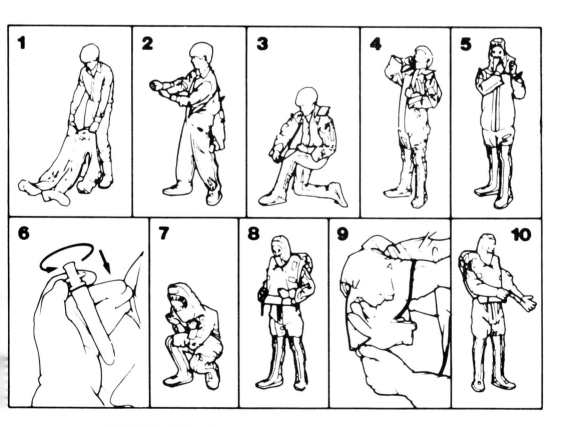

DONNING INSTRUCTIONS FOR A TYPICAL IMMERSION SUIT

Courtesy: Strentex Fabrics Ltd

# HAMMAR | H20

The Hammar H20 hydrostatic release unit consists of a double looped rope line, a release mechanism, and a weak link (red). The Hammar H20 is designed for liferafts carrying from 4 up to approximately 90 persons. It does not need servicing but MUST BE REPLACED AFTER TWO YEARS.

The Hammar H20 fulfils the requirements of the IMO-resolution A521 and the 1983 Amendments to SOLAS 1974. D.O.T. (UK) approved.

## INSTALLATION

The Hammar H20 is supplied complete including a weak link. The whole unit must be installed in accordance with the manufacturers instructions. The installation is simple and should be fitted as illustrated in the sketch and according to the following:

1. Check the unit for proper marking of year and month of expiry. PLEASE NOTE THAT THE UNIT HAS TO BE CORRECTLY MARKED TO BE ACCEPTABLE TO THE VARIOUS MARINE AUTHORITIES.

2. The Hammar H20 is to be installed with a shackle to a strong point on the deck or on the cradle. The shackle shall be fed through the thimble containing the "weak link" and the lower loop of the attachment line.

3. Fit another shackle through the larger loop of the attachment line and the upper loop of the weak link. The painter line of the liferaft shall also be secured to this shackle.

4. Install the liferaft in its cradle by means of a securing strap and senhouse sliphook. Attach the sliphook to the upper loop of the attachment line and firmly secure the liferaft.

## RELEASE DEPTH

The Hammar H20 will release the liferaft at a water depth between 1.5 and 4 meters.

The liferaft will float to the surface and the stretched painter activate the inflation of the liferaft. The weak link will break freeing the liferaft from the sinking vessel.

## MANUAL RELEASE

If the liferaft is to be launched manually the sliphook should be released and the liferaft thrown overboard. The raft is now attached to the vessel by the painter line and the Hammar H20 attachment line. Pulling the stretched painter line will inflate the raft and the survivors can board.

## THIS NOTICE MUST BE PLACED ABOARD THE VESSEL IN A CONSPICIOUS POSITION ADJACENT TO THE LIFERAFT STOWAGE.

## HYDROSTATIC RELEASE UNIT FOR LIFERAFTS

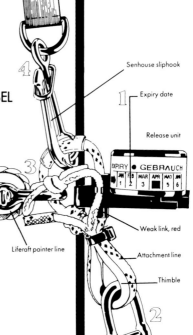

Senhouse sliphook

1 — Expiry date

Release unit

EXPIRY ● GEBRAUCH
JAN | FEB | MAR | APR | MAJ | JUN
1 | 2 | 3 | 4 | 5 | 6

Weak link, red

Liferaft painter line

Attachment line

Thimble

HYDROSTATIC RELEASE INSTALLATION INSTRUCTIONS

Courtesy: C. M. Hammar

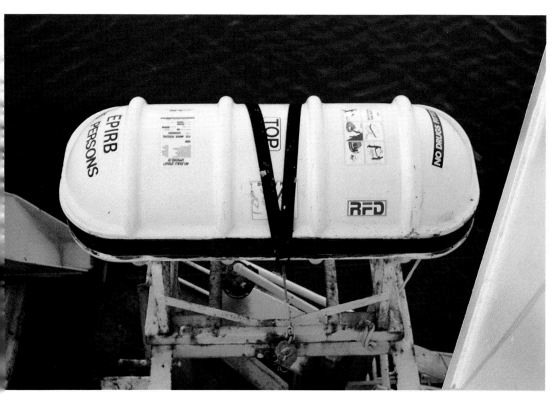

INFLATABLE LIFERAFT IN FIBREGLASS CONTAINER

Davit-launched liferafts are enclosed in fibreglass ontainers or canvas valises. Valises are stowed in ockers or boxes near the liferaft davit, and must be laced so that any lifting ring is uppermost. Rafts in ontainers are secured by hydrostatic releases, either ndividually or as a group.

The painters of inflatable liferafts should be secured ) the ship via the hydrostatic release at all times. In ne event of the ship sinking the raft will then float off, ulling the painter out of the container and inflating ne raft automatically when the end is reached.

A rigid liferaft is stowed on a wooden platform, rotected by a fibreglass cover which incorporates an utomatic release system that allows the liferaft to float ee if the ship sinks. The liferafts should be located ery close to or on a line with the ship's sides and it is nportant that there is enough room around each iferaft to allow the cover to open fully and let the iferaft float free. The cover is attached to the wooden latform by two nylon retainer straps which are clipped ) lugs on one side, and also by low breaking-strain ubber straps passed over hooks on the two adjacent

sides. Additional heavy weather lashings with a hydrostatic release may be fitted over the cover.

If a ship sinks before a rigid liferaft can be launched the liferaft will float free as follows:

- A hydrostatic release will free any heavy weather lashing.
- The buoyancy of the raft will break the rubber straps and attempt to lift the cover.
- The cover will turn over being restrained on one side by the nylon straps.
- As the cover turns over the raft will swing clear, float up, and rise to the surface.

*Note:* A rigid liferaft is operational no matter which way up it floats after launching. The lower canopy will fill with water and will act to reduce the rate of drift.

The painter system for both rigid and inflatable liferafts must incorporate a weak link or other device to ensure that a raft cannot be dragged down by a sinking ship. On certain older rafts the painter patch is arranged to tear away, on others a weak link is incorporated in

5

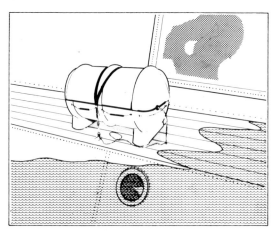

SINKING SHIP TAKES
LIFERAFT DOWN

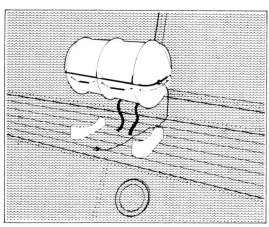

AT A DEPTH OF APPROX.
3 METRES HYDROSTATIC
RELEASE IS ACTIVATED &
LIFERAFT STARTS TO FLOAT
TO SURFACE.

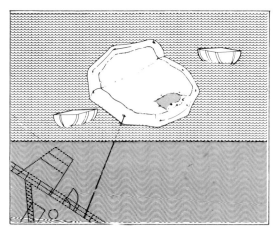

AS SHIP SINKS, PAINTER PAYS
OUT TO FULL EXTENT AND
ACTIVATES GAS CYLINDER TO
INFLATE LIFERAFT.

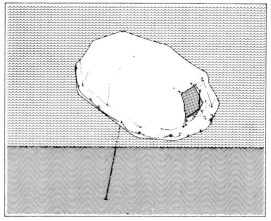

IF SHIP CONTINUES TO SINK
THE PAINTER OR A WEAK
LINK WILL PART AND THE
LIFERAFT WILL FLOAT CLEAR.

FLOAT FREE LAUNCHING OF INFLATABLE LIFERAFT

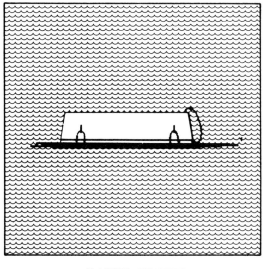

1) VESSEL SUBMERGED

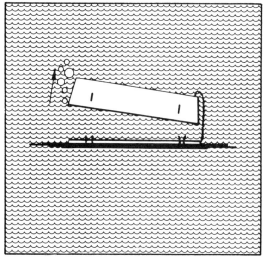

2) BUOYANCY OF RAFT BREAKS RUBBER
STRAPS, LIFTS COVER, WHICH, BEING
RESTRAINED ON ONE SIDE BY NYLON
STRAPS, STARTS TO TURN OVER.

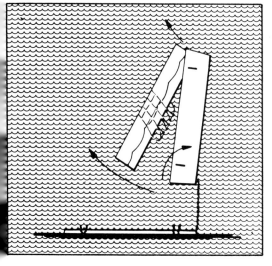

3) WHEN COVER HAS TURNED OVER THE
RAFT SWINGS CLEAR AND RISES TO
THE SURFACE.

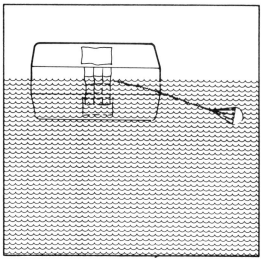

4) RAFT READY FOR BOARDING. CANOPIES
ARE RAISED AUTOMATICALLY BY PULLING
ON PAINTER OR CANOPY RELEASE LINE.

FLOAT-FREE LAUNCHING OF RIGID LIFERAFT

the painter itself or in the hydrostatic release. Where the weak link is incorporated in the painter it would normally be necessary, during a 'normal' abandonment and immediately after the raft has been launched, to secure the raft again using the 'strong' section of the painter to ensure the weak link does not break and allow the raft to blow away unloaded. In all cases those in charge of liferafts aboard ship should ensure that they have their painters and hydrostatic releases properly secured and fitted in accordance with the manufacturer's instructions.

## Rescue boats

Many older and all new ships are fitted with a rescue boat. These are mainly intended for rescuing anyone who falls overboard; they are also used to muster and tow liferafts and should be launched, if practicable, when abandoning ship.

Rescue boats may be of rigid or inflated construction, or a combination of both. If not of rigid construction they must always be fully inflated. Rescue boats may have an inboard engine or an outboard motor. Arrangements for towing liferafts are permanently fitted.

*Note:* A life boat may be constructed and fitted so that it fulfils the requirements of a rescue boat.

## Lifeboats

Lifeboats on older Australian ships are the standard open boats made of steel, aluminium or fibreglass, although totally enclosed fire resistant lifeboats have been supplied to some tankers, drilling ships and some recent cargo ships. New cargo ships, however, have totally enclosed lifeboats or, if operating in suitable areas, self-righting partially enclosed lifeboats.

Each lifeboat must have a separate set of davits. These are usually gravity davits although some ships use luffing davits. Some ships, under 500 gross tons, have one boat only with a davit system to put it into the water on either side of the ship.

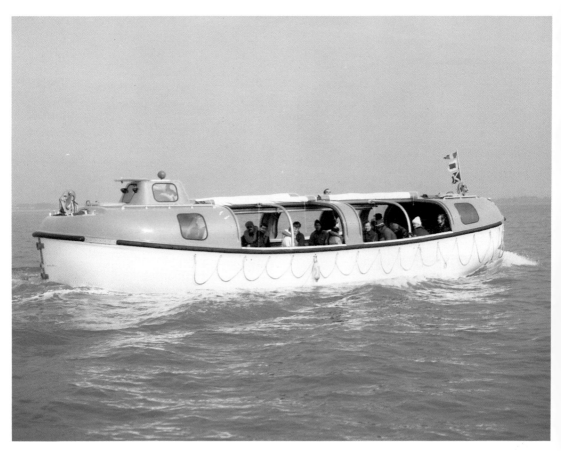

PARTIALLY ENCLOSED LIFEBOAT

Courtesy: Watercraft Ltd

Gravity davits are davits in which the swinging out and lowering of the lifeboat to the embarkation deck is accomplished by gravity once a restraining brake is released. Such davits come in two general forms: a roller trackway type, where the davit arms supporting the lifeboat are mounted on rollers which travel down inclined tracks; or a pivot type, where each davit is pivoted around a point inboard of the lifeboat so that the weight of the boat causes a turning out motion when the brake is lifted.

Luffing davits are davits which are turned outwards on a worm gear or screw.

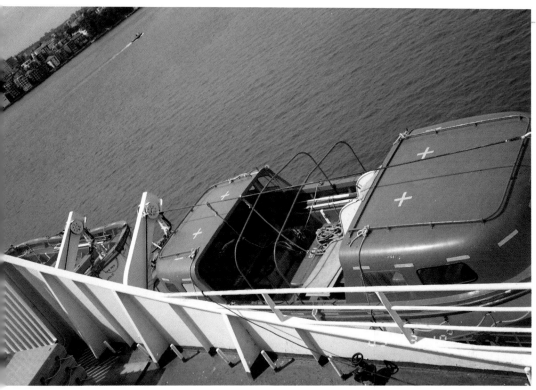

OPEN AND PARTIALLY ENCLOSED LIFEBOATS HUNG IN GRAVITY DAVITS
Courtesy: Cunard Line Ltd

Some cargo ships and oil rigs are fitted with stern launched free-fall lifeboats. These boats are totally enclosed and are designed to be launched 'free-fall' over the stern with their full complement. The lifeboat can also be lowered by gravity under manual control. A hydrostatic release may be incorporated in the arrangement, enabling the boat to float free after the ship sinks.

The most significant advantage of a free-fall lifeboat is the speed by which it can be launched and cleared from the ship. These boats can be hoisted on board in one continuous operation, from the water to the stowed position on board, by a separate single suspension system.

Lifeboats are normally served by wire rope falls and winches. At least two lifelines are fitted to the davit span wire between each pair of davits. However, totally enclosed lifeboats need not be fitted with lifelines. All lifeboats, other than emergency boats on passenger ships and stern launched lifeboats, must have skates to prevent them fouling projections on, or recesses in, the ship's side as they are launched. On some ships and oil rigs, lifeboats can be released and lowered from inside the lifeboat.

Lifeboats using gravity davits must have tricing pennants where it is necessary to bring them against the ship's side at the embarkation deck to load crew and passengers. Such lifeboats must also have bowsing

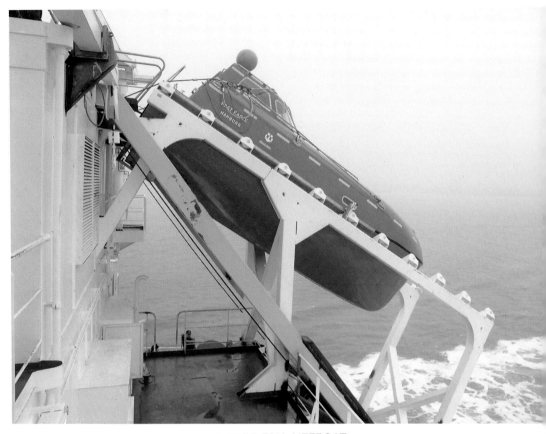

A FREE-FALL LIFEBOAT
Courtesy: Robert Hatecke Stader Bootswer

tackles or lines to ease them away from the ship's side before being lowered into the water. Tricing pennants and bowsing tackles or lines are unnecessary where people board lifeboats at the stowed position. On new cargo ships the full complement of a lifeboat must be able to board it at the stowed position in three minutes.

Totally enclosed lifeboats are self-righting. However, this can only be achieved if all the people in the boat are restrained in their seats with the seat belts provided and all entrances and openings are closed water tight. The buoyancy of a totally enclosed lifeboat must be such that, if holed in any one place below the waterline, there is no other damage, and no buoyancy material has been lost, it will support its full complement of people and equipment. Furthermore, it must have sufficient stability so that if capsized while damaged it will automatically position itself to provide an above-water escape for its occupants.

Totally enclosed lifeboats on tankers are fitted with a water-spray and a self-contained air support system.

## Survival capsules

Survival capsules are presently carried only on drilling rigs. The concept is similar to that of the totally enclosed and fire-resistant lifeboat, but with a circul or near-circular shape.

The capsule shell is made from fire retardant, gla reinforced plastic externally coloured international orange. The dome has two hinged access doors — o on each 'bow', a hatchway at the top, windows, ventilating manifolds, a fire sprinkler system, handrai and a hoisting/lowering hook. The capsule with equipment on board weighs approximately 2.3 tonne

Internally, a seat and a seat belt is provided for ea person the capsule is certified to carry, together wit compartments for food, water, tools and survival equipment. The survival capsule is fitted with a dies engine, bilge pump and lighting.

A davit system is being developed to carry them ships but at present on drilling rigs they are stowed

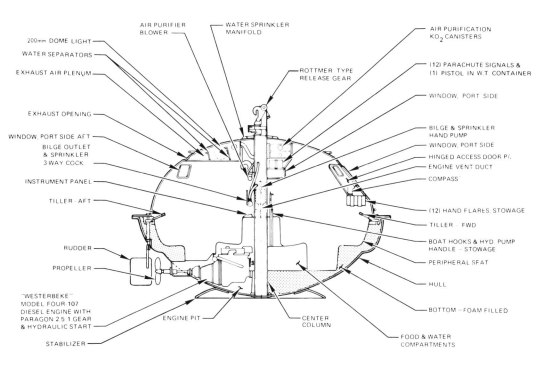

AIR PURIFIER BLOWER
WATER SPRINKLER MANIFOLD
200mm DOME LIGHT
WATER SEPARATORS
EXHAUST AIR PLENUM
ROTTMER TYPE RELEASE GEAR
EXHAUST OPENING
WINDOW, PORT SIDE AFT
BILGE OUTLET & SPRINKLER 3 WAY COCK
INSTRUMENT PANEL
TILLER - AFT
RUDDER
PROPELLER
"WESTERBEKE" MODEL FOUR-107 DIESEL ENGINE WITH PARAGON 2 5 1 GEAR & HYDRAULIC START
STABILIZER
ENGINE PIT
CENTER COLUMN
AIR PURIFICATION KO_2 CANISTERS
(12) PARACHUTE SIGNALS & (1) PISTOL IN W.T. CONTAINER
WINDOW, PORT SIDE
BILGE & SPRINKLER HAND PUMP
WINDOW, PORT SIDE
HINGED ACCESS DOOR P/L
ENGINE VENT DUCT
COMPASS
(12) HAND FLARES, STOWAGE
TILLER - FWD
BOAT HOOKS & HYD. PUMP HANDLE - STOWAGE
PERIPHERAL SEAT
HULL
BOTTOM - FOAM FILLED
FOOD & WATER COMPARTMENTS

## WHITTAKER SURVIVAL CAPSULE

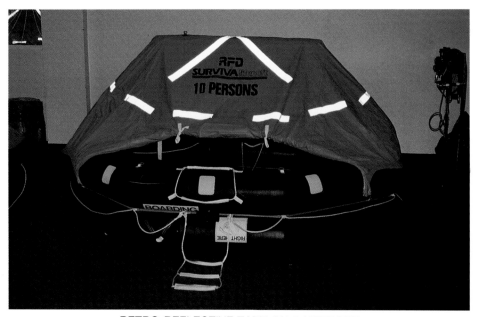

## RETRO-REFLECTIVE TAPE ON A LIFERAFT
Courtesy: RFD Safety Marine P/L

11

under a holding platform which extends outboard over the water. They are lowered automatically on a single wire after all personnel have boarded and a winch release handle above the upper hatchway has been pulled from inside the capsule.

### Retro-reflective tape

Retro-reflective material reflects any light shone on it from a torch, signal lamp or searchlight. The following items of life-saving appliances are fitted with retro-reflective tape: lifeboats, survival capsules, rescue boats, liferafts, buoyant apparatus, lifebuoys, lifejackets, immersion suits and thermal protective aids.

### Emergency Position Indicating Radio Beacons (EPIRBs)

All large commercial ships carry a 406 MHz EPIRB, which must be stowed so as to float free if the ship sinks. If time permits, this EPIRB should be placed in one of the survival craft before abandonment. A crew member should be specifically assigned this task in the muster list.

Each liferaft contains an EPIRB operating on 121.5/243 MHz. These EPIRBs are particularly useful for searching aircraft to locate survival craft.

### Radar reflectors and transponders

Each liferaft contains either a radar reflector or a radar transponder. Where radar reflectors are stowed in each survival craft, a radar transponder must be stowed each side of the ship, so they can be rapidly placed in any survival craft. Two crew members should be assigned this task in the muster list. Radar reflectors and transponders enhance the detection of survival craft from searching ships.

### Two-way radiotelephone apparatus

All ships must carry portable marine VHF transceivers (two-way radios) for communication between survival craft, between survival craft and ship, and between rescue boat and ship. At least three are required on each ship.

### Ship's parachute distress signals

All ships carry 12 parachute distress rockets, similar to the rockets provided in survival craft, to attract the attention of searching aircraft or ships. These rockets are stowed in a clearly marked distress signal locker which is usually located in or close to the navigation bridge.

### Ship's line-throwing apparatus

Most ships are equipped with a rocket line-throwing apparatus capable of throwing a light line over a distance of 230 metres. The apparatus can be used to send a line to another ship or to the shore to prepare for the rescue/retrieval of survivors and survival craft

There are four rockets and four lines, or four self-contained units (each containing a rocket and line ready for use). Before firing a rocket to a tanker, check that it is safe to do so.

## ORGANISATION AND TRAINING

Dealing efficiently with an emergency situation should be the aim of all personnel on an Australian ship, both as individuals and as the crew of the ship. Preparation for such a situation is a matter of knowledge and experience which can be gained from information on the ship and from practising the use of life-saving and emergency equipment at practice drills. Films, lectures and discussion groups are also very useful.

The revised Chapter III of SOLAS 74 (1983 amendments) sets out the basic requirements for the organisation and training required on a ship. These are summarised below.

### Muster lists

Muster lists are posted where they can be easily read such as the navigating bridge, engine room and crew accommodation. They give details of the General Emergency Alarm Signal and how the Abandon Ship Signal is to be given. They also show the duties assigned to each member of the crew, which officers are assigned the duty of ensuring life-saving and fire-fighting appliances are maintained in good order ready for use, and specify substitutes for key personnel in the event of their being disabled.

On passenger ships a notice giving the muster station of the occupant or occupants is exhibited in each passenger cabin. Illustrated instructions for donning lifejackets are also displayed in each cabin and at passenger muster stations.

### Emergency signals

The General Emergency Alarm Signal is seven or more short blasts followed by one long blast on the ship's whistle or siren.

The Abandon Ship Signal will be specified on the muster list and may be a verbal command, a supplementary signal on the general emergency alarm system, or it may be given by other suitable means.

Signals will be repeated on the ship's electrically operated warning bell system and suitable instruction given on the public address system or by any other effective means available.

## Musters and drills requirements

| | |
|---|---|
| Muster of passengers on a passenger ship engaged on an international voyage | Within 24 hours after the passengers have embarked |
| Drill of the crew of a passenger ship | Weekly, and on an international voyage, prior to the ship leaving the final port of departure |
| Drill of the crew of a ship other than a passenger ship | Monthly, and within 24 hours after the ship leaves port where more than one quarter of the crew has been replaced |
| Abandon ship and rescue boat drills | Monthly |
| Liferaft drill | Every three months |
| Fire drill | Every month |

## Conducting musters and drills

The master of a ship must ensure that personnel are trained in the handling and use of the life-saving appliances and are thoroughly conversant with the duties assigned to them. It is vital that practice drills be carried out as realistically as possible. Their purpose is to ensure that every person on board knows the emergency signals, knows what to do, and is trained so that this is done efficiently. Where practicable some drills should be conducted after dark, using emergency lighting only.

Ships' masters must take a dominant interest in drills. They must see that all personnel attend and that the drills are carried out realistically. The minimum legal requirements are listed in the appendices to Marine Orders Part 29, and in corresponding State/Territory legislation. Times of drills should be varied so that no crew member is excused from two consecutive drills. Duties when swinging out and launching survival craft should be varied so that all personnel get practice. Lifejackets must be inspected to see that they are worn and tied correctly. Everyone must know how to activate the lifejacket light. Each crew member must study any posters or notices about life-saving equipment and ask if in doubt about any equipment or how it is used.

## VITAL KNOWLEDGE FOR CREW MEMBERS

*Crew members must ensure they know:*
- *where lifejackets are and that they are ready to put on and are not lashed up in a ball;*
- *how to put them on correctly and operate the light;*
- *the duties assigned to them;*
- *the location of the survival craft on the ship and how to launch such craft;*
- *the escape routes from working and accommodation areas to the emergency stations and to the survival craft embarkation areas;*
- *the Emergency and Abandon Ship Signals.*

# Chapter 2
# Abandonment

This chapter covers the operations required for the breaking-out, launching, disengagement and clearing away of survival craft with a full complement of persons.

## CONTENTS OF THIS CHAPTER

## THE ORDER 'ABANDON SHIP'

The order to abandon ship must only be given at the express command of the master or person in charge of the ship, and then only where the ship is in such distress due to collision, fire, explosion or other cause that the lives of the people on board are endangered. Timing the order to abandon ship is of great importance as it signifies the end of attempts to save the ship.

As long as the ship continues to float and there is a safe or relatively safe area for people on board, including escape routes to survival craft, the ship should not be abandoned. The ship is the best survival unit and is more easily found by searching aircraft or ships.

The order to abandon ship would be expected to follow after:

- an incident, e.g. collision, fire, explosion;
- sounding of the General Emergency Alarm Signal for the muster of crew and passengers at their emergency stations;
- operations of the collision-damage party, fire-fighting parties, etc.;
- making of Urgency and/or Distress Signals;
- the possible arrival of rescue or stand-by ships.

Crew members are trained through practice drills for these situations.

Where circumstances do not allow this order of events, the best use should be made of any time available to make a Distress Signal, muster everyone on board, and prepare survival craft. Generally the smaller the ship the less time there is between a disaster and abandoning ship, resulting in a 'crash' abandonment. It is essential that the crew are familiar with the location of immersion suits, lifejackets, lifebuoys and all survival craft on board.

The Abandon Ship order is to be specified on the muster list. Ideally, the order should be given verbally, using the ship's telephone or loud-speaker system. Every possible attempt must be made to pass the order to every person on board. This order may be supplemented on the General Emergency Alarm System with a signal of distinctive character. A signal comprising three 'A's in Morse Code ($\bullet - \bullet - \bullet -$) would be an appropriate example. Before giving the Abandon Ship Signal all isolated parties should, if possible, be warned to withdraw in good order and proceed to their allotted survival craft. This may be done by word of mouth, over the public address system or portable radios, via messengers, or by putting the engine room telegraph at 'Finished With Engines'.

Ringing 'Finished With Engines' is not a signal to abandon ship, but it indicates that abandonment is imminent. On receipt of this telegraph order crew members should stop or make safe all machinery that could hamper abandonment, or be a hazard to life during abandonment, if this has not already been done. This could include stopping pumps with an overside discharge in way of survival craft, stopping main engines and propellors and retracting stabilisers.

## PREPARING AND LAUNCHING SURVIVAL CRAFT

### After General Emergency Alarm Signal given

The master of an Australian ship is required to assign particular duties to each crew member to be carried out if an emergency occurs. These special duties include equipping lifeboats and other life-saving appliances, preparing survival craft for launching and preparing other life-saving appliances for use.

It is essential for safe abandonment that those people assigned to the special duty of preparing survival craft for launching should go immediately to their emergency stations and begin their duties on hearing the General Emergency Alarm Signal.

Unless a direct command to the contrary is given by the master, they should prepare lifeboats for launching (lowering them to the embarkation deck, if they are not boarded from the stowed position), prepare liferafts for launching and, where davit-launched liferafts are carried, hook on the first liferaft at each station ready for inflating. Lifeboat and liferaft embarkation ladders should be made ready. Portable radio equipment, first-aid kits, narcotic drugs, two-way radiotelephone apparatus, and additional equipment for survival craft (see page 21 for a suggested list of additional equipment) should be put into survival craft.

The person in charge of a survival craft should ensure that the overside discharges have been shut. Stabilisers, if fitted, could interfere with the safe launching of the survival craft and the person in charge of the survival craft should make sure that the stabilisers are withdrawn before launching.

### Personal preparation before abandoning

Loss of body heat is one of the greatest hazards faced by seafarers forced to abandon ship. The rate of heat loss depends on the ambient temperature, the protective clothing worn and the way the seafarer conducts himself or herself when in the water. Many ships, especially small ships, sink in less than 15 minutes after the emergency is discovered.

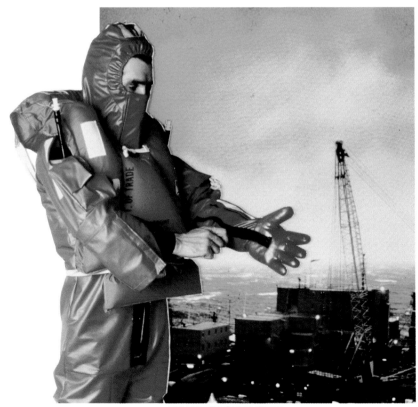

AN IMMERSION SUIT

Courtesy: Strentex Fabrics Ltd

15

Remember to:

- Put on as much warm clothing as possible making sure that head, neck, hands and feet are covered.
- Replace heavy boots or shoes by soft soled footwear such as sandshoes.
- Put an immersion suit on over warm clothing if one is available.
- Unless the immersion suit is also your lifejacket, put on a lifejacket and secure it properly.
- Take anti-seasickness tablets. (Vomiting loses essential water and seasickness makes a person prone to hypothermia.)
- Drink as much water as possible.
- Avoid getting into the water if possible.
- Avoid jumping into the water — the shock of sudden immersion in cold water can kill.
- Button up your clothing, turn on your lifejacket light (at night) and put the whistle in your mouth as soon as possible before your hands go numb.
- Get out of the water as soon as possible.

## After Abandon Ship order given

When the order to abandon ship is given all crew members should proceed to their survival craft embarkation areas. Passengers, if any, will already have been mustered and accounted for and should be led to the embarkation areas by those crew members appointed to this task. It is essential that the person in charge of each survival craft should check the attendance of each person allotted to it.

Passengers and crew should board the survival craft in an orderly fashion and crew members with special duties for the launching of the craft should take up their correct positions. They should then launch the survival craft unless the Abandon Ship order has been countermanded or other instructions have been received.

## Lifeboats

*Gravity davits, lifeboats embarked at an embarkation deck*

- Send toggle painter well forward outside all obstructions until the slack is taken up and secure aboard ship.
- Check that davit locking pins are out.
- Let go gripes (check that triggers have fallen).

- Lower to embarkation deck until tricing pendants bring boat alongside, but do not allow the full weight of the boat to come on the pendants. Make fast bowsing-in ropes or tackles. Ship rudder and tiller, and insert drain plugs. Flake lifelines ready for lowering, so they will not foul the boat or occupants on lowering.
- Let go tricing pendants.
- Wait for order to embark (place additional equipment and supplies in lifeboat, and start engine).
- Embark passengers and crew (women and children first, all to be seated as low as possible).
- Ease off bowsing-in ropes or tackles and let go.
- Lower boat (land boat on crest of wave so that drop into trough will overhaul falls, and ensure brake stays off till falls are unhooked). Unhook falls (after fall first, then for'd fall if making headway).
- Embark launching party via embarkation ladder in calm weather. In rough weather boat should clear ship's side as soon as possible. When the boat is clear the launching party should climb down the ladder or jump, and swim to the boat. It will help them if the end of the buoyant line has been passed round the bottom rung of the ladder so they can pull themselves to the boat instead of having to swim.
- If vessel is making way, spring off. Otherwise push off. Let go or cut toggle painter.
- Clear the ship, and if not motor boat, stream sea anchor or drogue. If motor boat, assist other craft clear of ship, group them together and pick up survivors from water.

*(SEE NOTES A AND B, p. 20)*

*Gravity davits, lifeboats that can be embarked at the inboard (stowed) position*

- Send the toggle painter well forward until the slack is taken up and secure aboard ship.
- Check that davit locking pins are out.
- Ship rudder and tiller and insert drain plugs.
- Place additional equipment and supplies in lifeboat.
- Embark passengers and crew.
- Let go gripes (check that triggers have fallen).
- Lower boat.

The rest of the procedure is as for 'Gravity davits, lifeboats embarked at an embarkation deck'.

### Where ship is equipped with luffing davits

- Send toggle painter well forward until the slack is taken up and secure aboard ship.
- Let go gripes and turn down any chocks (lift boat clear if necessary).
- Turn out the davits.
- Lower to embarkation deck.
- Turn in davits to bring boat alongside and make fast bowsing-in ropes or tackles. Ship rudder and insert drain plugs. Flake lifelines ready for lowering.
- Wait for order to embark (place additional equipment and supplies in lifeboats).
- Embark passengers and crew (all to be seated as low as possible). Ease off bowsing-in ropes or tackles and let go. Turn out davits to full extent.

- Lower lifeboat.

The rest of the procedure is as for gravity davits. *(SEE NOTE C, p. 20)*

### Where ship is equipped with free-fall lifeboats

- Remove portable rails/safety chains if any and gripes.
- Enter lifeboat, be seated in the boat and fasten seat belts. (Failure to properly secure seat belts could lead to severe injury; accelerations up to 6g may be experienced.)
- Coxswain to check all openings are closed, start engine, warn of imminent launch.
- Activate the free-fall control and the lifeboat will slide down the ramp and drop in the water clear of the ship.

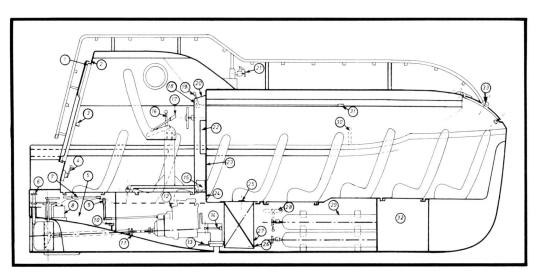

GENERAL ARRANGEMENT FOR FREEFALL-LIFEBOATS

| | | |
|---|---|---|
| (1) socket for charging battery | (12) emergency stop | (23) socket for emergency transmitter |
| (2) searchlight | (13) shutoff valve sprinkler pump | (24) earthing for transmitter |
| (3) holder for antenna | (14) coupling sprinkler pump | (25) to filled fuel tank |
| (4) manual pump | (15) battery charger | (26) drain cock |
| (5) equipment | (16) engine control lever | (27) fuel valve |
| (6) hydraulic jack with release bolt | (17) hydraulic pump for release bolt | (28) charging valve for air bottles |
| (7) emergency tiller | (18) air pressure gauge | (29) air bottles |
| (8) battery | (19) valve for compressed air | (30) hook to lash |
| (9) spring starter | (20) switchboard | (31) compressed air exit |
| (10) stern tube greasing | (21) wash-line sprinkler connection | (32) drinking water and equipment |
| (11) stuffing box | (22) holder for emergency transmitter | (33) ventilator lockable |

**GENERAL ARRANGEMENT FOR A FREE-FALL LIFEBOAT**
**Courtesy: Robert Hatecke Stader Bootswerft**

- The crew will withstand the impact without injury provided they are seated and properly secured with seat belts. In the event of a capsize the boat is self-righting, again provided all occupants are secured. The boat may also be launched by the recovery davit or crane. However, in an emergency the free-fall method will always be used by reason of time. The recovery davit or crane *may not be designed to handle a fully laden boat.*

*(SEE NOTE D, p. 20)*

## Inflatable liferafts (*throw over*)
- Remove any lift-out railings or safety chains.
- Check painter made fast on board. Operate hydrostatic release and remove securing strap.
- Lower any ramps or guides for projecting liferaft outboard. Await orders for launching.
- Check water below launching point is clear and throw or roll liferaft overboard.
- Pull remainder of painter out, and give a hard tug to fire the gas bottle.
- Raft inflates in 20 to 30 seconds. Pull raft alongside on painter.

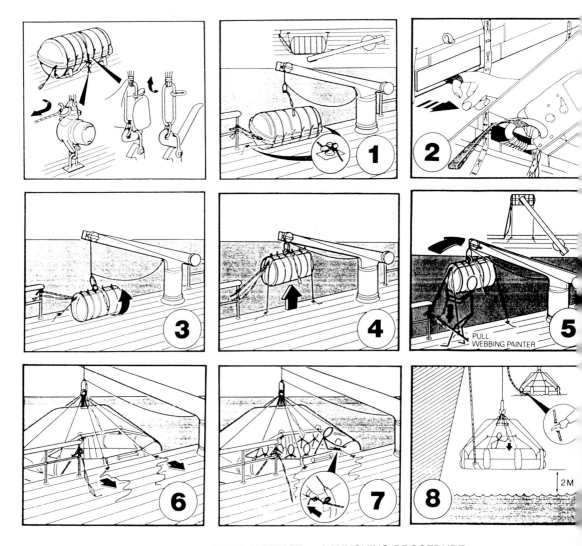

**DAVIT LAUNCHED LIFERAFT — LAUNCHING PROCEDURE**

Courtesy: RFD Limited

- If necessary put one person in water or, preferably, direct onto the raft to right a liferaft which inflates upside down. Do not delay as righting a capsized raft tethered by its painter in strong winds is difficult if not impossible. If raft cannot be righted while tethered it may be necessary for all crew to enter water, swim to raft, cut painter, right raft and then board. Inflated rafts subject to wind will blow away from ship's side and in strong winds may capsize or break away. Do not delay in manning raft after inflation.
- Board liferaft using embarkation ladder if possible. Remove shoes and sharp objects and try to avoid injury to persons in the raft if it is necessary to jump into the raft. Jumping is very undesirable except onto an empty raft.
- When all persons are on board cut the painter as far away from raft as possible. (Knife stowed in pocket near painter.)
- Paddle clear of ship and join other craft. Stream the sea anchor or drogue.
- If 'blow off' valves are inside the raft, ventilate to remove $CO_2$ from atmosphere in raft.
- Commence removing water from inside raft. Inflate floor.
- Keep look out for survivors and other rafts.

## Davit-launched liferafts
- Remove railings at launching station. Slew davit outboard keeping hook secured inboard.
- Bring liferaft from storage. Position raft and attach bowsing-in lines to cleats.
- Attach hook to suspension link and lock hook.
- Await order to inflate liferaft and secure for embarkation. Bring up other rafts from storage.
- Raise the fall to put liferaft outboard, and then inflate raft.
- When liferaft fully inflated adjust bowsing lines and inspect raft. With two people tending entrance, embark personnel commencing to seat them alternately forward and aft, with later persons on either side of first persons with feet towards centre. (Remove shoes and all sharp objects from persons before boarding.)
- When raft is loaded release bowsing lines and check water below launching point is clear.
- Lower away. On raft pull red lanyard to operate the hook safety catch as the raft nears the water.
- The hook will release itself when raft is waterborne. Retrieve hook for next launching.
- Launching crew hold painter while raft is launched then, if conditions are appropriate,

secure it to next raft when ready. Secure painter of last raft launched to ship to hold raft near ship while launching crew descend ladder and swim to raft. Then cut painter.
- Clear raft from ship with paddles to join other craft. Stream the sea anchor or drogue.

### Alternative procedure where practical
Slew davit inboard above inflating point. Position raft, inflate when ordered, hook on while passengers and crew board raft. Lift, then slew davit outboard and lower. Retrieve hook and repeat for next raft.

## Rigid liferafts
- Release heavy-weather straps.
- Remove cover and plastic sheeting.
- If necessary, move raft to a position for launching.
- Remove any lift-out railings or safety chains.
- Await orders for launching. Check painter made fast on board ship.
- Check water below launching point is clear and launch raft.
- Pull on painter, and tug hard to erect both liferaft canopies. Pull raft alongside with painter and board using embarkation ladder if possible. Remove shoes and sharp objects and try to avoid injury to persons in the raft if it is necessary to jump.
- When all persons are on board, cut the painter as far away from the raft as possible (knife stowed near painter).
- Paddle clear of ship to join other craft. Stream the sea anchor or drogue.

## Other survival craft

### Rescue boats
- Attach lifting bridle and hook on.
- Fit outboard motor and fuel tank (if carried) to rescue boat.
- Raise boat clear of chocks.
- Swing boat outboard and lower to embarkation level. Lead painter well forward and secure aboard ship so that painter will be taut before rescue boat touches water (essential if vessel has headway).
- Start engine (some engines or motors should not be started without cooling water) and await instructions for launching.

- Embark crew.
- Lower away.
- Release bridle. Let go painter.
- Manoeuvre rescue boat to clear ship and prepare to tow liferafts clear.

*Survival capsules*
- Release securing hooks.
- Open capsule doors and top hatch.
- Wait for order to embark, start engine.
- Embark personnel through both doorways, moving to outboard seats. Close doors. Ensure personnel strapped in seats.
- Operate lowering control. Operate air purification system in oil fire or heavy weather.
- Release hook when craft waterborne.
- Clear ship. If necessary operate sprinkler system.

*NOTE A:* For fully enclosed lifeboats lowering is controlled from inside the boat. In an oil fire or heavy weather the launch is 'closed up' with an air support system operating. Operate the sprinkler system in an oil fire. It is essential for all personnel to use the safety belts provided as these craft are not self-righting unless everyone is strapped in.

*NOTE B:* Pre-1986 lifeboats may have lifeboat fall disengaging gear permitting simultaneous off-load release (that is, when boat is fully waterborne). Post-1986 lifeboats are required to have disengaging gear permitting simultaneous release both off-load and on-load (that is, when boat is fully waterborne, or when weight of boat is partly or fully on the falls). Crew members are advised it is essential that these types of disengaging gear be maintained in strict accordance with the manufacturer's instructions and tested at least every three months, and crew members should be trained in their use, including operation of the device to protect against accidental or premature use. Whilst post-1986 lifeboats are designed to withstand a fully laden drop of three metres into the water the on-load release capability *should only be tested when the boat is waterborne.*

*NOTE C:* When lowering all lifeboats to the embarkation deck it is important that gripe wires do not foul the lifeboats or davits, that people in the boats sit down and hold onto lifelines and that the full weight of the boat is not allowed to come on the tricing pendant. Bowsing-in ropes or tackles should be rigged with the hauling parts in the boat.

This last point may not be possible with totally enclosed boats.

*NOTE D:* Should the ship sink with an unmanned lifeboat, a hydrostatic release or releases incorporated in the system may allow the lifeboat to float free.

## When no emergency signal given ('crash' abandonment)

There are instances when a sudden disaster occurs to a ship which, despite the best intentions of the people on board and the most rigorous training, puts the ship into such a state of distress that immediate abandonment is necessary. Such occurrences may include collision, sudden shift of cargo, explosion, sudden impact damage to underwater hull, or a combination of these factors. The smaller the ship the quicker disaster can overwhelm it.

Training for situations where first indications of distress immediately precede the order to abandon ship cannot be easily met. Shipboard training will normally be directed towards the situation where an Emergency Signal is given, although priorities must be considered for a crash abandonment. Generally, if the crew members are adequately prepared for emergencies, any abandonment will be more likely to be successful.

### Priorities for 'crash' abandonment
- Make 'Abandon Ship' Signals by all means and to all parts of ship. Ship's engines should be stopped.
- Send 'Distress Message' by ship's communication equipment.
- Muster all persons. Check lifejackets worn.
- Launch as many survival craft as possible.
- Move portable radio equipment to survival craft or throw into water to be retrieved.
- Abandon and clear away from ship.
- Look for retro-reflective tapes and lights on other lifesaving appliances, and look and listen for other survivors.

## IMPORTANT CONSIDERATIONS WHEN ABANDONING SHIP

### Passengers

In an emergency situation on a ship where passengers are carried, a decision must bemadewhether the passengers would be safer if they remain on the ship or if they are embarked in urvival craft. The course of action to follow will depend upon factors such as the:

* type and location of hazard to ship;
* probability of continuing success of operations against that hazard;
* safety of survival craft and their embarkation points;
* sea and weather conditions;
* approach of rescue or stand-by ship.

Early abandonment by passengers may not be warranted when the crews of lifeboats or other urvival craft to which passengers are assigned would have to be withdrawn from firefighting, collision or other emergency duties.

## Early launching of survival craft

On any ship in a distress situation, it may be necessary to launch survival craft at an early stage. This is particularly so in ships with fires in accommodation or hatch areas adjacent to the embarkation points for survival craft. Alternatively, liferafts could be moved to parts of the ship remote from fire or collision damage.

As far as possible liferafts should not be inflated until required. Liferaft containers or valises should be placed in lifeboats which are to be cleared away from the ship or should be placed in the water to be towed clear by lifeboats or rescue boats. Should abandonment not be necessary appliances can then be replaced on board.

Where ships are in collision and/or are likely to take a severe list, attempts should be made at an early stage to launch at least the lifeboat(s) from the high side of the ship and, if possible, some liferafts as an insurance against difficulties in abandoning ship at a later stage.

## Additional equipment for survival craft

Where there is time between preparing survival craft for launching and abandonment, efforts should be made to obtain additional equipment useful in survival craft.

The following items are suggested and could be towed ready for use in suitable locations:

extra water — fill clean containers to three-quarters capacity. These will float and can be towed by survival craft;

ship's pyrotechnics;

sweet biscuits, fresh and dried fruits, tinned and bottled fruit juices and soft drinks;

* blankets and additional clothing;
* battery-operated Aldis signalling lamp (unsealed acid or alkaline batteries should not be taken into an inflatable liferaft);
* additional torches, batteries and bulbs;
* notebook and pencil for keeping a log;
* ship's charts of area marked with ship's estimated position, and a current chart;
* sextant, chronometer, almanac and tables;
* palm, needles and twine;
* sunscreen or similar anti-sunburn ointment, if available;
* oilskins and waterproof material, e.g. tarpaulins, plastic sheeting;
* extra fuel and oil for motor lifeboats to be towed in same manner as water;
* non-mineral oil, such as fish oil or colza oil;
* light rope for towing purposes;
* buckets; and
* protection for the head such as beanies or other headgear to help reduce loss of body heat.

The above list is in addition to the radar transponders, the float-free EPIRB, the two-way radios, and drugs which are required to go into the survival craft.

Obviously the size and number of survival craft dictate the amount of additional equipment to carry. A non-passenger ship with 200 per cent lifeboat capacity and 100 per cent liferaft capacity should be able to find plenty of room in lifeboats for additional equipment.

If time permits, everyone abandoning ship should drink plenty of water and take anti-seasickness tablets. To be most effective these should be taken 30 to 60 minutes before abandonment, but when this cannot be done they should be handed out by the person in charge who calls the roll at each survival craft.

## Using all survival craft in abandonment

When abandoning a ship equipped with both lifeboats and liferaft, the lifeboats should be regarded as the primary survival craft provided that they can be launched safely. However, every attempt should be made to launch liferafts and to tow them, either inflated or non-inflated, clear of the ship. Alternatively, they can be retrieved when they float to the surface. Liferafts that have not been inflated should not be towed by their operating painters.

Where several liferafts can be towed clear in this manner, the equipment of the rafts should be used before that of the lifeboats. In particular, the Emergency Position Indicating Radio Beacons (EPIRBs) MUST be obtained from the liferafts, which are the only survival craft in which they are carried.

*Where a ship can be abandoned using all survival craft and the craft can be grouped together, the availability of fresh water and stores is greatly increased. This means a similar increase in the expected survival time.*

### Lighting arrangements for launching survival craft

Ships are provided with means for illuminating:
- alleyways, stairways and exits to facilitate access to the stowage and launching stations of the various survival craft;
- survival craft and their gear, during their preparation for and in the process of launching;
- the area of the water into which the survival craft are to be launched.

Power for the illumination is provided by the ship's main power supply and also by the emergency source of power.

Where an additional liferaft is carried in the forward or after end of the ship, illumination is provided by an emergency light or an electric torch which is stowed near the liferaft. Torches provided on tankers are required to be intrinsically safe.

### Availability of ship's position

To expedite sending a distress or urgency message a reasonably up-to-date ship's position should always be available to the radio officer or radio telephone operator. GMDSS communications equipment should be supplied with accurate position and time information at least once a watch.

The ship's position, actual or estimated, should be noted at least every watch, and preferably at intervals of two hours, together with details of ship's course and speed.

This information should also be given to those in charge of survival craft when abandoning ship, together with direction and distance of nearest land.

### Marine Evacuation System (MES) launching and embarkation

On ships where a marine evacuation system is provided, the evacuation slide is to be under the charge of an officer, or a person with a Certificate of Proficiency in survival craft.

People leaving the ship by MES should muster at the muster station, and follow the instructions of the person in charge.

## SURVIVAL IN THE WATER

### Righting a liferaft

When an inflatable liferaft inflates upside down it may be righted in the following manner:
- Pull raft around until the gas bottle is downwind.
- Get onto inverted floor of raft.
- Set feet on gas bottle, then heave raft over by pulling on righting strap.

When an inflated raft is capsized the buoyancy of the arch tubes or centre strut will oppose the capsize until overcome by the weight of water entering the canopy. The sooner therefore the raft can be righted the easier the operation will be. See comments on righting capsized rafts on page 19.

### Jumping into survival craft

Whenever possible survival craft should be boarded before they are lowered, or directly from the embarkation ladders. If it is necessary to jump onto them, care should be taken to avoid jumping onto people already in the survival craft. Shoes and sharp objects should be removed before jumping. Jumping should be avoided if at all possible.

### Jumping into water

If it is necessary to jump into the water, jump from the lowest possible point and then swim to survival craft. If you have to jump, keep your elbows to your side, cover nose and mouth with one hand while holding the wrist or elbow with the other hand. Ensure that your lifejacket is correctly and securely tied before jumping. Should the danger of the ship capsizing or sinking appear imminent, persons should jump from the bow or stern of the ship, provided in the latter case that the propeller has been stopped. It is always preferable to climb down a ladder, a rope or even a fire hose.

### Dangers due to cooling in water

Sea water temperatures depend largely on latitude and season. In most areas of the world immersion in the sea will cause cooling of the body, which is normally at a temperature of 37°C.

The great enemy of a survivor in the water is hypothermia. Hypothermia means lowered, deep-body temperature (see page 55 for a discussion of hypothermia). In cold water the skin and peripheral tissues become cooled very rapidly, but it takes 10 to 15 minutes before the temperature of the heart and brain begins to fall. Intense shivering occurs in an attempt to counteract the large heat loss.

The graph on page 24 shows predicted survival times of average, adult humans in water of different temperatures. The figures are based on extrapolation of experimental cooling rates of average men and women who were holding still in ocean water and wearing a standard lifejacket and light clothing. The graph shows, for example, that the predicted survival time is less than three hours in water of 10°C. None of the 1489 persons immersed in 0 degree Celsius water at the sinking of the *Titanic* in 1912 was alive when rescue vessels arrived 1 hour 50 minutes later; almost all those in lifeboats survived.

Although the body produces almost three times as much heat when swimming slowly and steadily (e.g. side stroke) as when holding still, this extra heat, and more, is lost to the cold water due to increased blood circulation to the arms, legs and skin. An average person in a lifejacket cools 35 per cent faster when swimming than when holding still. Survivors should not attempt to swim except to stay afloat, move away from a sinking ship or get to a survival craft. The average person in water 10°C is unable to swim 1.5 km before being incapacitated by the cold.

In the water a survivor without a lifejacket is forced to adopt some 'anti-drowning' behaviour as few people can hold their heads for long above water while remaining motionless. The following method may be used.

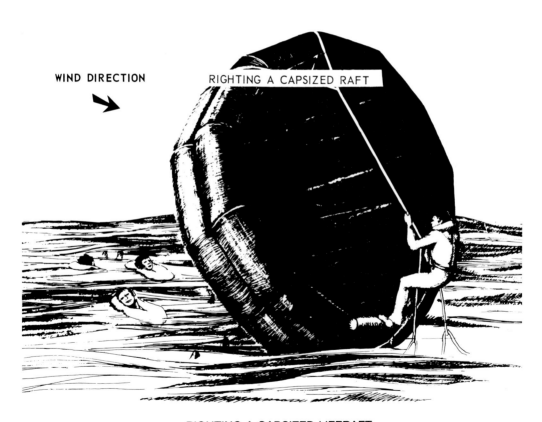

WIND DIRECTION

RIGHTING A CAPSIZED RAFT

RIGHTING A CAPSIZED LIFERAFT

### Treading water

Continuous movement of arms and legs in certain patterns keeps the head out of water. This may be enhanced by breathing in deeply and holding the breath as long as possible, and only treading water while breathing out and in.

Treading water is the preferred method as others involve putting the head (a high heat loss area) into the water, thus increasing the cooling rate.

### HELP — Heat Escape Lessening Posture

A survivor in a lifejacket is in a much better situation as he or she can remain motionless with the head out of the water and can adopt a better position to retain body heat — the Heat Escape Lessening Posture (HELP).

The inner sides of the arms are held tight to the sides of the chest and the thighs are raised to close off the groin region. The head is above water. This posture gives an increase in predicted survival time of nearly 50 per cent.

### The 'Group Huddle'

Where several survivors are in the water together their survival will be enhanced if they form a ring facing towards the centre and linking arms close together. This is known as the 'Group Huddle'. The water inside the ring is calmer than outside, lessening the adverse effects of wave splash, and lessening the heat loss on one side of the body.

Survivors should not discard clothing while in the water unless it is absolutely necessary. Most clothing does not decrease buoyancy significantly and added layers of clothing decrease the rate of body cooling, thus enhancing survival time. Even boots and shoes, when worn with socks, probably are on balance preferable to bare feet or socks alone.

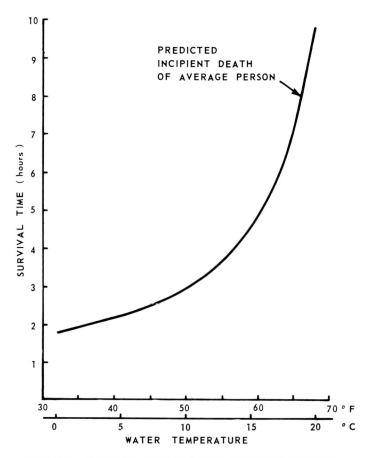

MAXIMUM SURVIVAL TIME IN COLD AND WARM WATER

The following table gives the predicted survival time for a lightly clothed adult in water of 10°C.

| Situation | Action/behaviour | Predicted survival time (hours) |
|---|---|---|
| No lifejacket | Drownproofing (not recommended) | 1.5 |
| No lifejacket | Treading water | 2.0 |
| Lifejacket | Swimming | 2.0 |
| Lifejacket | HELP | 4.0 |

Survivors should make use of any floating wreckage to raise themselves out of the water (even partially).

*Consumption of alcohol before entering the water results in an increased cooling rate and hastens death.*

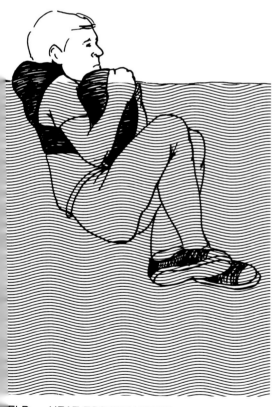

ELP — HEAT ESCAPE LESSENING POSTURE

## IMMEDIATE ACTION AFTER ENTERING SURVIVAL CRAFT

Irrespective of the type of survival craft, there are six basic steps for immediate action.

1. Get away from the sinking or burning ship.
- Let go toggle painter or cut painter as far from raft as possible.
- Manoeuvre or drift to a safe distance. In a totally enclosed lifeboat, or a survival capsule, once well beyond an oil fire on the sea surface the hatchways can be opened and the water spray and air support systems, if in use, can be shut down.
- Stream sea anchors in a liferaft when well clear.

2. Look for and gather survivors.
- Use torches at night to spot reflections from retro-reflective tape.
- Listen for whistles.

    In motor boats, rescue boats or capsules, use the engine, in other lifeboats use the oars, in rafts use the paddles — to get to survivors in the water.
- In rafts use rescue quoits and lines to pull survivors to the raft.

3. Join other survival craft.
- Look for survival craft lights.
- Use motor boats, survival capsules, rescue boats and oar propelled lifeboats to gather survival craft together.
- Secure all survival craft together using remains of painters on rafts with as long a drift as possible. Allow room for movement in a seaway.
- Stream sea anchors or drogues.

4. Check for proper functioning of the survival craft.
- Check for damage, leaks, fire damage. Plug air leaks on an inflatable raft with leak stoppers from the equipment bag.
- Top up buoyancy chambers if necessary with pump or bellows.

5. Begin measures for protection and survival.
- Erect canopies on lifeboats.
- Inflate floor on liferafts.
- Give first aid to injured.
- Take action against seasickness (if not done before abandoning ship).
- Take steps to retain body heat of persons who have been in water.

6. Read survival manual again.

# Chapter 3
# Survival instructions

This chapter is concerned with keeping people alive until rescued.

These instructions cannot and do not attempt to cover everything which may happen to people in survival craft. They do, however, advise survivors of the basic actions and information necessary for their continued safe existence in lifeboats or liferafts.

Survivors who read these instructions must determine their relevance in view of the circumstances at the time. Such factors as sending distress signals, approaching rescue craft and the closeness of the coastline should be taken into account when deciding what action to take.

## CONTENTS OF THIS CHAPTER

## THE INITIAL SITUATION — IMMEDIATE ACTION IN SURVIVAL CRAFT

Immediately after abandoning ship and entering the survival craft survivors are likely to be cold, wet, possibly exhausted from fire-fighting etc., and suffering from varying degrees of shock. Mental and/or physical let-down leading to collapse is a possibility, but must be resisted until the situation of all survivors is consolidated.

Every effort should be made to complete the 'Immediate Action' instructions. The person in charge of each survival craft should decide the order in which these actions are carried out. Many actions may be taken concurrently, for example: rescuing survivors in the water, joining the survival craft together, treating the injured and preventing seasickness.

Some actions are of greater importance than others in this initial phase, such as rescuing survivors from the water and gathering the craft together to increase the chances of detection. Measures for the protection and comfort of the occupants can follow later.

### Need for immediate artificial respiration

People in charge of survival craft should know that a lack of oxygen to the brain for three to four minutes can be fatal, as the body's vital organs and nerve centres will be affected. Where apparently drowned survivors are recovered from the water *artificial respiration must begin immediately* and be continued whatever the other actions or movements of the craft or of survivors in the craft. See instructions for cardio-pulmonary resuscitation on page 50.

### Lookout duties

The 'Immediate Action' duties are to look (and listen) for survivors in the water and to look for other survival craft. Lookouts should look and listen for:

- lifejacket lights
- lifebuoy lights
- lights from other survival craft
- retro-reflective tapes on lifejackets, lifebuoys and other craft

- gas 'blow-off' from inflatable liferafts
- whistles from survivors in water
- shouts from survivors in water
- passing ships and aircraft

This phase ends when all survivors have been picked up from the water, and when no other isolated survival craft can be seen. However, the lookout's duty to watch for ships and aircraft continues until the survivors are rescued (see pages 45 and 60–61).

## Rescuing survivors in water

When survivors are seen in the water but the survival craft cannot manoeuvre towards them, the rescue quoit and line or the buoyant heaving line or lines should be thrown towards them. If necessary a person from the survival craft, preferably a strong swimmer wearing a lifejacket, should swim to the survivors taking the end of the heaving line or lines. This should be a voluntary action.

People in the water should preferably be taken into lifeboats over the weather bow or quarter, and helped into liferafts. Where injured people in the water are taken into a liferaft they should (when possible) be turned with their backs to the raft, and held by one person on each side with one hand on the shoulder and the other below the armpit. The survivor, depending upon injuries and the risk of inhaling water or oil on the water, should first be pushed down to obtain a boost from natural buoyancy and buoyancy of any lifejacket, then lifted up and slid over the buoyancy tube on the survivor's back.

Depending on the numbers involved, it may be desirable that survivors should first be gathered to the survival craft and then taken on board. People in the water clinging to survival craft should tie themselves on or put arms through lifelines on the craft rather than hold on with hands which might become numb and let go.

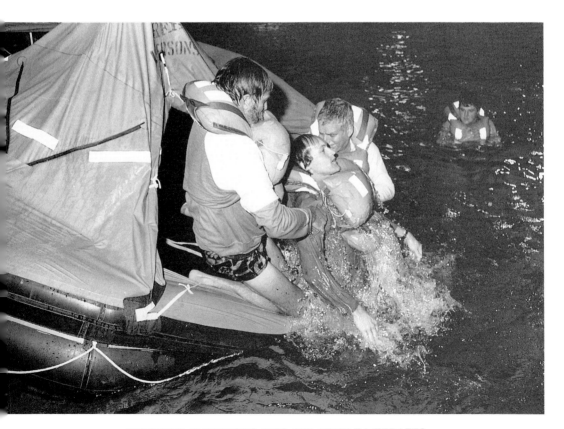

ASSISTING SURVIVORS INTO INFLATABLE LIFERAFTS
Courtesy: Australian Maritime College

27

## Gathering and securing survival craft together

Gathering together survival craft is best carried out by motor lifeboats or rescue boats and, to a lesser extent, by lifeboats under oars. When this is not possible, assembling liferafts may be done by varying the speed downwind of the rafts and by movement across wind. If drogues are not streamed, an inflatable liferaft will drift very quickly at about two or three times the rate of liferafts with drogues streamed.

A method of moving liferafts across the wind, or moving liferafts in calm seas is by 'kedging' with the drogue or sea anchor. Tie a weight to the drogue and throw the drogue and weight as far as possible in the direction required; allow the drogue to sink and then pull the liferaft up to the drogue. Repeat this action as required.

Rigid liferafts, with the lower canopy acting as a form of drogue, will drift at a slower rate than inflatable liferafts.

When survival craft have been gathered together, they should be made fast by enough length of doubled lines to allow for wave action. A suitable length of line for rough weather is about 10 metres. Avoid joining craft together by short lines as wave action will jerk and pull on lines, possibly damaging painter patches, etc., or may snatch at rafts, allowing the wind to get underneath to capsize them.

When joining craft together lifeboats should be to windward because of superior sea anchors. They can also spread suitable oil from the oil bag if one is aboard the lifeboat to flatten the seas around themselves and the liferafts.

## Distributing survivors and equipment among survival craft

Where survival craft have grouped together, the most senior person should consider the arrangement of survivors among the various craft.

Where survival craft are all liferafts, transferring people from one raft to another can be carried out to equalise the numbers in each liferaft. In warm weather the fewer the number of people in each raft the cooler they will be.

In cold weather it may be preferable to keep rafts up to full complement to raise the temperature inside to aid retention of body warmth. Any additional rafts should be kept available for possible later use.

In liferafts survivors should be spaced out evenly, sitting with feet towards the centre and arms through handlines secured inside rafts to give support and to reduce the possibility of rough weather tipping the liferaft over. Wearing hard-soled footwear in 10-person or smaller rafts can be very uncomfortable for other occupants when the raft is full. Hard-soled footwear should be removed but retained for later use.

The atmosphere inside an enclosed liferaft can become uncomfortably warm and humid even with a relatively cold outside atmosphere. Occupants in the raft should resist the urge to remove their clothing. In such circumstances it is advisable to open the flaps and ventilate the liferaft as necessary.

## Inflatable liferaft functions

During the initial inflation, the relief valves on the liferaft buoyancy chambers will 'blow off' excess gas after normal pressure is obtained. The valves should then be fitted with the plugs supplied (these are stowed in the equipment bag) to prevent dirt and sea water getting in. These plugs should be removed several times during a hot day to allow the raft to 'blow off' and should be removed whenever the buoyancy chambers are to be 'topped up' by use of the pump or bellows.

Whenever the raft 'blows off' or if a leak occurs in a buoyancy tube the raft should be ventilated to disperse the gas. Where leaks occur leak stoppers should be inserted as a temporary repair. Use the smallest leak stopper that will do the job and screw it in sufficiently to plug the leak but not so far that it will increase the size of any hole or tear. Survivors entering inflatable liferafts should, of course, remove all items likely to damage the rafts, such as shoes, buckles, rings, knives or pieces of wreckage.

## Preserving body heat

When survival craft are clear of the abandoned ship and, preferably, have gathered together, it is essential to start taking measures to protect survivors.

All persons whose clothing is wet from immersion in water or from sitting in water in survival craft should remove their clothing, wring it as dry as possible, and put it back on. It is not easy for this to be done, particularly in inflatable liferafts, and care must be taken to avoid upsetting the craft or other people. Movements should be kept to a minimum and cooperation is required.

If possible, at the same time, attempts should be made to pump or bail out the survival craft and dry all areas where survivors are sitting or lying using the sponges provided or cloths. This may seem a futile task in rough weather but must be continued to reduce the risk of hypothermia, immersion foot and salt water sores. The weather side in particular should be closed off, if possible, in order to keep the craft dry.

HOT WEATHER – MAXIMUM VENTILATION AND FLOOR DEFLATED

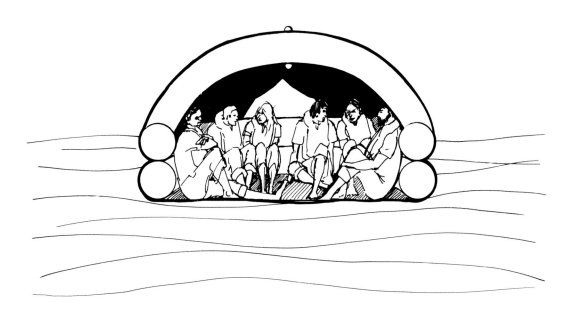

COLD WEATHER – MINIMUM VENTILATION AND FLOOR INFLATED

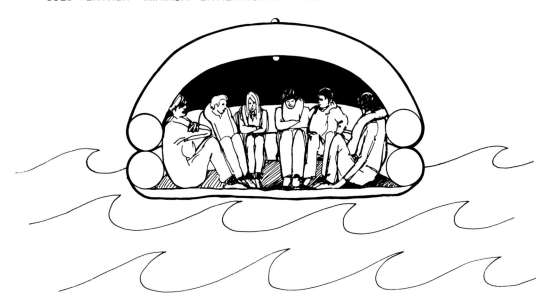

PROTECTION FROM HEAT AND COLD IN INFLATABLE LIFERAFTS

Generally, clothing should be shared between survivors but special care should be taken of the sick and injured. Waterproof or windproof clothing should be worn by those doing lookout duty or otherwise on watch in the open.

Once the survival craft has been dried out as much as possible, efforts should be made to raise the body temperature of survivors. This action is vital in cold weather or when survivors have had prolonged immersion in water.

In liferafts the canopy entrances should be closed and survivors should huddle together for warmth. In inflatable liferafts the floor should be inflated. The body heat alone of occupants will raise the temperature inside the raft and maintain such temperature. Tests in sub-zero temperatures have demonstrated that the temperature inside a liferaft can be raised to 16°C in an hour in this way.

The situation in enclosed lifeboats and survival capsules is very similar to that in the liferaft. Providing hatchways are closed and ventilation reduced to a minimum, the inside temperature can be raised.

The least protection against cold is offered by the open lifeboat, where windchill can also be a factor. However, the use of exposure covers reduces windchill. Both ends of exposure covers need closing before the temperature inside the cover can be raised by the occupants.

Where survivors are taken from the water after prolonged immersion, action to regain body heat should be started immediately. For the first 20 minutes out of the water the body core temperature of survivors will most likely continue to drop. Survival depends on the actions described above and on warmth given by people already in the survival craft.

## Preventing seasickness

Tablets to prevent seasickness are carried in all survival craft. These should be issued to all survivors for the first two days, whether or not they feel seasick. The movements of small survival craft, particularly where occupants are enclosed by canopies, exposure covers, etc., are very likely to lead to outbreaks of seasickness, even for people who have never been affected before.

As well as causing distress, vomiting causes a loss of valuable moisture from the body which must then be replaced. People affected by seasickness should attempt to fight the lethargy induced by it while there is urgent work to be done.

Place vomiting people near an entrance. This should be a priority, as fresh air will reduce seasickness.

## Beginning first aid treatment for the injured
*(See first aid instructions)*

Generally, the treatment of injured survivors should begin as soon as possible after the survival craft has cleared away from the abandoned ship. It is obviously better for people qualified in first aid to give such treatment, and where survival craft can be quickly gathered together either the 'first aider' or the 'patient' should be transferred to the same craft, depending on the nature of the injuries.

Where a survivor is apparently drowned or asphyxiated, mouth to mouth resuscitation must be started at the earliest possible time.

## ORGANISING EVENTUAL SURVIVAL

To achieve eventual survival it is essential that routine duties be carried out by the occupants of a survival craft. Organising and performing such duties are boost to the morale of survivors.

Organisation among a group of survivors is best achieved when there is one person in charge of each survival craft. Where ship's officers are present they would be expected to take command of the craft, unless incapacitated. Where no officers are present, a senior crew member should take charge. If there is no obvious leader the survivors in each craft should choose a leader and be aware that their choice indicates acceptance of the leader and agreement to obey instructions.

The leader of a survival craft, whether by rank or by being chosen, must have a knowledge of the survival craft and its use. The leader would normally be the holder of at least a Certificate of Proficiency in Survival Craft or a Lifeboatman's Certificate.

The rules for survival are mainly a matter of commonsense. The leader of a survival craft should ensure above all that the will to live and the means to live are maintained, while not neglecting the location and possible detection of the craft.

The 'means to live' consist of the survival craft and its equipment and rations. Maintaining these requires the performance of the following duties: maintaining the survival craft, medical duties, issue of rations, and supplementing rations.

The 'will to live' is strengthened by organising a routine for the above duties, and for lookout, navigation, and record keeping.

The 'will to live' is also increased by knowledge of the survival craft and by appreciating the conditions likely to be encountered. Within the limitations of the survival craft's size, and of reducing physical exertion to the minimum to avoid an increased need for water, survivors should be kept physically and mentally busy.

Allocating duties will vary according to the size of the survival craft and the number of occupants. Duties must be carried out around the clock, involving setting up some form of watch system. The need for rest and sleep should not be forgotten.

In a six-person liferaft, for example, some duties might be shared by two people at a time (i.e. lookout and raft maintenance, with a third survivor 'on call' for collecting rainwater, treating injured, etc.). Rations could be issued at the change-over of watches, and a watch-and-watch-about system will be necessary.

In a lifeboat or large liferaft a three or four-watch system might be possible, with six or more people to a watch so that all occupants are involved in the duties. More than one person may then be allocated to perform certain duties. Where possible the 'lookout' should be changed at frequent intervals, particularly in very cold weather. The duties should be rotated where possible during each watch to avoid undue physical exertion.

The greatest danger to achieving survival is fear and panic resulting from ignorance of the correct use of survival craft. Leaders of survival craft containing passengers must impress on them the safety provided by the craft if the required duties are carried out and must involve them in such duties.

At the earliest possible time the leader of each craft should attempt to record the circumstances leading up to abandonment of the ship, and account for as many persons as possible. Each occupant of the craft should be questioned about actions taken, people sighted and not sighted, etc.

If possible a log should be kept of the time in the survival craft. This should contain details of duties organised, rations issued or supplemented, first aid treatment, the condition of the craft and condition of each survivor.

Where survival craft have been gathered together organising for survival is easier. The senior person present will take charge of all the assembled craft. This allows certain duties to be concentrated in the larger craft and particularly in the lifeboats, where less maintenance is required.

If possible injured people should be grouped together for attention, depending on the state of their injuries and the advisability of moving them.

Where survival craft have been gathered together the use of the various means to attract attention becomes subject to the instructions of the senior person present, ensuring better use of the signals and avoiding the simultaneous use of two signals or Emergency Position Indicating Radio Beacons (EPIRBs).

Pooling together is good for morale as the chances of being detected are increased, while for the smaller manned liferafts the performance of duties is eased. Raft maintenance then becomes the prime duty rather than keeping a lookout.

## MORALE

When people are packed together tightly their behaviour changes. It is important that people do not annoy each other. If there appears to be a problem it must be corrected as soon as noticed. If necessary persons should be transferred between craft to minimise friction. Special care should be taken in establishing a proper procedure for the normally private acts of urination and defecation.

One of the greatest problems for survivors is to fill in the time when not carrying out the allocated duties. This manual should be read by all survivors and can form a basis for discussion. People in charge of survival craft should ensure that the use of playing cards does not lead to gambling for food or water rations or to bad feeling among the survivors.

Survivors should only be allowed to smoke providing great care is exercised with matches and cigarettes, and providing other occupants do not object at times when the entrances are closed. Smoking may exacerbrate thirst and should not be allowed when the water supply is low.

Depending on water supply and the dryness of throat and mouth of survivors, morale may be sustained by singing, by prayer, by discussions on the achievement of survival, and by telling jokes, stories, and so on.

## MAINTAINING SURVIVAL CRAFT

To achieve survival it is essential that each survival craft performs all the intended functions throughout a life-saving incident. These functions will vary slightly according to the type of craft, but generally consist of:

- retaining buoyancy
- protecting occupants
- using the drogue or sea anchor
- lighting the survival craft, and
- securing the craft together.

### Retaining buoyancy

*Survival craft are required to be buoyant.*

The buoyancy tube or tubes of an inflatable liferaft should be inspected frequently for leaks and damage. Impact damage to the buoyancy tube will result in rapid deflation, so temporary repairs must be made as soon as possible with the use of leak stoppers and the buoyancy tube pumped up again.

A slow deflation is likely to be caused by pinhole leaks which may be difficult, if not impossible, to find, especially if below water level.

Generally, temporary repairs should be made good as soon as possible, using the repair kit in the raft. It is easier to patch the raft if the area is dry in preparation for the solution, although it is possible to patch areas under the water. When making permanent repairs any patch should extend at least 25mm outside the damaged area.

Even if the buoyancy tubes are not leaking or damaged, they will need attention throughout each day. The sun's heat will expand the gas in the raft during the day, and the plugs must be removed from the relief valves to allow any excess pressure to 'blow off' Consequently, each evening after the sun has set the buoyancy tubes will become flabby and must be inflated by using the pump or bellows. Arch tubes or centre strut tubes should be treated in the same manner.

### Protecting occupants

Protecting occupants from exposure to heat or cold is a major function of survival craft. Protection is provided by canopies, which may be either rigid or fabric.

Rigid canopies are fitted to totally enclosed lifeboats and survival capsules. These canopies are fitted with hatchways and doors for access and for extra ventilation in hot weather.

All open lifeboats are equipped with exposure covers which can be rigged by survivors in the boats. These covers are usually supported on frames or hoops and extend from the bow for 70 per cent of the length of the lifeboat, giving slightly less than one metre

headroom above the thwarts and side benches. Crews should be practised in rigging these beforehand.

New cargo ships have totally enclosed boats but if they only trade in suitable areas they may have partially enclosed boats. These are also allowed on new passenger ships. Partially enclosed boats have a combination of rigid and permanently attached folding covers; crews should be practised in their erection.

The rigid cover extends from both bow and stern of the lifeboat for at least 20 per cent of the length of the boat in each case; the folding cover encloses the remaining length of the boat. Together the covers completely enclose the occupants in a weatherproof shelter.

These covers should be rigged as soon as possible after abandoning ship to protect survivors from the effects of windchill and from spray or rain. In hot weather the cover protects survivors against sunburn and the sides or entrances of the cover should be opened to increase ventilation. The after end of the cover on open boats should remain open to provide an escape in case the lifeboat capsizes.

As many survivors as possible should be protected by the cover, with the exception of people 'on watch'.

The 'Floating Igloo' rigid liferaft has a canopy with double walls on each side. Each canopy is provided with two openings which can be closed to keep out spray and wind. The lower canopy fills with water when the raft is launched and gives great stability to the raft.

The double skin of the canopies provides an insulation barrier and the canopy entrances can be closed to keep out the weather and yet maintain ventilation. The canopies are erected when the raft is launched by operation of spring loaded hoops or frames released by pulling on the painter line or by use of a canopy line.

Survivors in a rigid liferaft must not strain against the top of the canopy and must not disturb the canopy frames. A liferaft paddle should be used to support the middle of the canopy except when rain water is being collected. A pocket is supplied for the paddle blade when used to support the canopy.

Inflatable liferafts are also fitted with a double canopy to protect the occupants against exposure, the layer of air between the two canopies acting as an insulation barrier. The entrance or entrances to the liferaft are also double, with the outer canopy being lowered and secured to the top of the buoyancy compartment and the inner canopy being drawn upwards. The entrances to the raft can be closed to prevent sea water or spray entering the raft while still obtaining sufficient ventilation.

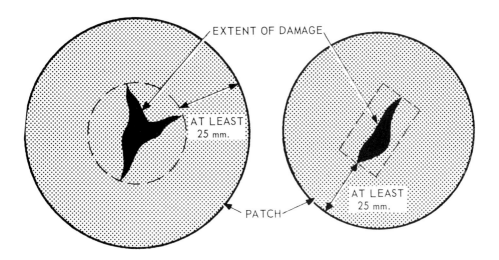

1) DRY OFF AND CLEAN DAMAGED AREA
2) APPLY ADHESIVE TO DAMAGED AREA AND PATCH
3) MATE SURFACES WHILE ADHESIVE IS STILL TACKY
4) SMOOTH OUT PATCH TO REMOVE AIR
5) LEAVE AT LEAST 30 MINUTES BEFORE RE-INFLATING

## USE OF PATCHES

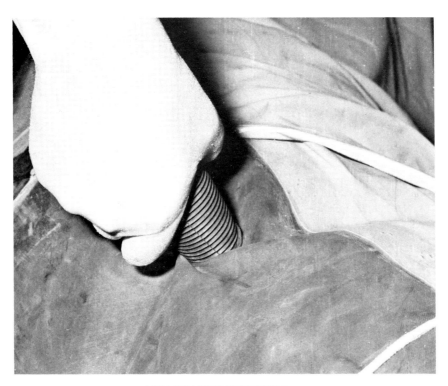

USE OF LEAK STOPPERS

REPAIRS TO INFLATABLE LIFERAFTS

As the entrances are secured by tapes or drawstrings it is essential that these are not overstressed, torn or cut, or tied in such a manner as to prevent their easy release.

It is not unusual for survivors to require maximum ventilation and cooling during the day — which may necessitate constant wetting of the canopy with sea water — and then to require maximum warmth in the liferaft during the night.

The floor of an inflatable liferaft can be inflated manually. Inflation of the floor is related to the sea temperature; generally the floor is inflated in cold weather as insulation against the cold water and deflated in hot weather to provide cooling. It is also suggested that survivors sit on their lifejackets or lay them out on top of the floor as a mattress for increased comfort and insulation.

Care must be taken when inflating or deflating the floor that the inflate/deflate valve is not damaged or the deflation probe lost.

### Using the sea anchor or drogue

Survival craft are provided with a sea anchor or drogue to reduce the rate of drift away from the abandon ship position, to reduce the likely search area.

A sea anchor streamed from a lifeboat will also keep the bow, or stern if preferred, up into the wind and sea and so reduce the risk of broaching to, or capsizing. The anchor or drogue of a liferaft is also important as it will prevent the liferaft from spinning round in circles and will hold it fairly steady relative to the wind.

Lifeboats are provided with a sea anchor complete with hawser and tripping line. Older lifeboats also have a can full of oil (usually fish oil or a light vegetable oil) and an oilbag. In rough seas the oil bag may be filled and streamed with the sea anchor to reduce the breaking of seas around the lifeboat and any attached craft. Lifeboat sea anchors are subject to severe strain in heavy weather. The hawser should be protected from chafe and inspected regularly. The tripping line allows the sea anchor to be 'tripped' for hauling in.

Liferafts are provided with a sea anchor or drogue attached to a strong point on the raft and lightly lashed so that it may be easily released as soon as required. A spare drogue is usually stowed with the other equipment. It is essential to use the drogue

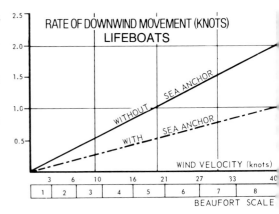

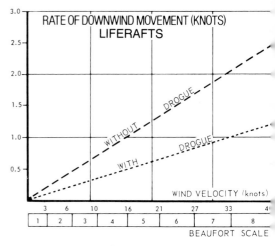

**DRIFT RATES FOR SURVIVAL CRAFT**

continuously, so the drogue and its line should be checked frequently for damage to the drogue materi bridle or line, or to the attachment point on the raft

Survivors in liferafts should be aware of the possibility of varying the point of attachment of the line to the raft (by lashing the painter around part of the raft's circumference) in order to gain more shel from heavy seas or to gain additional ventilation by altering the position of the raft openings relative to t direction of the sea anchor.

Should a sea anchor or drogue carry away, every attempt should be made to rig a jury sea anchor. In lifeboats a jury sea anchor can be made from masts and sails lashed together and streamed on a bridle secured to the hawser or to a painter. Where mast and sails are not carried, use two oars lashed together with any available material such as sea anchor bag, exposure cover bag or lifejackets. A temporary sea anchor can be made using two buckets and a buoyant line. With the bight of the line inboard, make each end fast to the handle of a bucket (and around the bucket, for safety), and pay out one bucket on each bow.

In liferafts, if both drogues are lost, every attempt should be made to rig a jury sea anchor using whatever is available on the raft, for example, paddles tied to lifejackets or discarded clothing, a pair of trousers with legs tied and the waist held open. If retained when the raft is inflated, the fibreglass container or the canvas valise could be used as an additional drogue.

No tripping line is provided for liferaft drogues. To increase the rate of drift the liferaft must be hauled up to the drogue, which must then be taken from the water. It may be necessary to increase the rate of drift in order to clear rocks or reefs, or to take advantage of an onshore breeze.

Survival capsules are not normally provided with sea anchors.

## Lighting survival craft

All survival craft are provided with inside lights for use when needed. Some of these lights may also be used as aids towards finding the craft.

An open lifeboat is equipped with an oil lamp and a torch with spare batteries and bulb. The oil lamp reservoir contains oil for 12 hours use, and an extra five litres of colza oil or kerosene is usually carried.

The oil lamp can be used for general lighting at night in the lifeboat, and for display on the approach of search aircraft or ships. The lamp must also be small enough to fit inside the two buckets provided in the boat, for use in flashing or signalling.

The torch should be used when searching for survivors in the water after abandoning ship and then restricted to attracting the attention of searching ships or aircraft.

Partly and totally enclosed lifeboats and survival capsules have battery-operated interior lights and a light mounted on the top of the cover or enclosure. In these craft any oil lamp (if available) should only be used outside the craft.

Inflatable liferafts are provided with exterior and interior canopy lights powered by a dry battery or a sea-water-activated cell. This latter cell is attached to the buoyancy tube below the water level and will become active as soon as the liferaft inflates, irrespective of the time of day.

If liferafts are launched in daylight there is no point in wasting the life of water-activated cells. Remove the cell from its pocket or strap, which should be done, if possible, without sending a person into the water although the cells are usually located well away from the canopy entrances. When the cell has been retrieved, the water should be vigorously shaken out and, if possible, placed or held in sunlight to aid drying out.

The chemical action in the cells will already have started so the full life will not be preserved, but some use will be gained from the cells when they are reshipped for the night and possibly some life may be left for the following night.

New rigid liferafts have lights similar to those on inflatable liferafts, the lights being activated as soon as the canopy is erected. Older rigid liferafts are not provided with lights fitted to their canopies, but have a battery-operated buoyant light attached to the raft by a lanyard. During the day this light should be retrieved and slung or stowed upside down to deactivate the battery.

All liferafts are provided with chemiluminescent lights and with torches. The chemiluminescent lights are intended for inside lighting only. The lights are activated by bending the light stick to break an inner phial and mix two liquids together, producing a greenish yellow light. Care must therefore be taken in handling unused light sticks and the movement of other equipment stowed with them. Each light stick will give three to four hours of reasonable light before fading, although total life of each light may be up to 12 hours. The light sticks can be easily handled and moved around the liferaft when operating.

Survivors should also be aware of the potential light source from lifejacket lights which have not been activated by sea water. Such lights should be removed from lifejackets and used for internal lighting, possibly by immersing the cell in a container of sea water in the craft. They may also be used to mark liferafts during the night after the expiry of the exterior canopy light.

## Securing survival craft together

Gathering and securing together survival craft is a major function for motor lifeboats and rescue boats. The second painter and the buoyant lines of lifeboats will most likely be the main source of lines for securing craft together. If the craft are secured close alongside use lifejackets or other items as fenders.

Where circumstances permit, survival craft should be secured together with enough line to prevent jerking and pulling due to wave action. The tow line or securing line should be made fast to a strong point of the raft and preferably be backed up to a second point.

Such lines should be inspected regularly for possible damage or deterioration, and particularly for any chafing where lines pass over lifeboat gunwales. Where possible a second line should be rigged as a stand-by to each craft.

Above all, the attachment points of lines to liferafts must be checked to ensure that towing patches or other strong points are not being torn or pulled away from the liferaft.

People in charge of motor lifeboats or rescue boats should be aware that if such securing lines fail they will have to 'round up' the free craft.

Survivors should also keep in mind the possible use of motor lifeboats, etc: to tow other survival craft clear of the abandoned ship or of points of danger, or to the shore if nearby.

## SURVIVAL CRAFT EQUIPMENT

### Liferaft equipment

| | | |
|---|---|---|
| Sea anchors | A | two, one permanently attached to the liferaft and one spare |
| Buoyant bailer | B | one, two for rafts larger than 12-person |
| Pump or bellows for topping-up raft (inflatable liferafts only) | C | one |
| Puncture repair kit (inflatable liferafts only) | D | one |

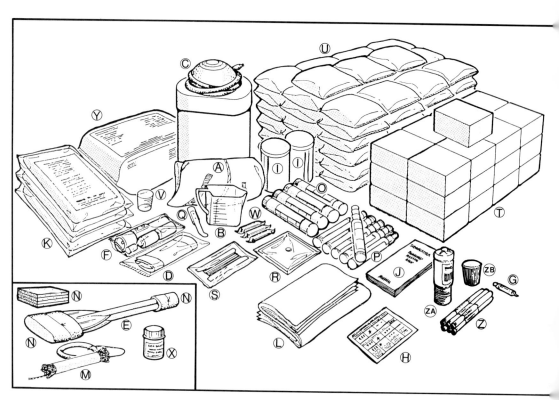

LIFERAFT EQUIPMENT

Courtesy: RFD Limited

| Item | | Quantity |
|---|---|---|
| Buoyant paddles | E | two |
| Waterproof torch | F | one, spare set of batteries and spare bulb |
| Whistle | G | one |
| A copy of the Rescue Signal table used by lifesaving stations, marine rescue units and ships and persons in distress | H | one |
| Buoyant smoke signals | I | two |
| Instructions for immediate action and instructions on how to survive | J | one copy of *Survival at Sea* |
| Thermal protective aid | K | two, three for 25-person rafts |
| Seasickness bag | L | one per person |
| Buoyant rescue quoit | M | one with at least 30 metres buoyant line |
| Sponges | N | one for each person |
| Parachute distress rockets | O | four |
| Hand flares | P | six |
| Safety knife | Q | one, two for rafts larger than 12-person |
| Heliograph | R | one |
| Fishing kit | S | one fishing line and six hooks |
| Food ration | T | Food giving at least 10,000 kilojoules for each person (approx 667g per person) |
| Water ration | U | 1.5 litres of fresh water for each person the liferaft is permitted to accommodate of which 0.5 litres may be replaced by a de-salting apparatus capable of producing an equal amount of fresh water in two days |
| Drinking vessel graduated | V | one |
| Tin openers | W | three |
| Seasickness tablets | X | six for each person, with instructions |
| First aid outfit | Y | one, in resealable watertight case |
| Chemi-luminescent lights | Z | six |
| EPIRB* | ZA | an Emergency Position-Indicating Radio Beacon |
| Matches | ZB | one watertight container |
| Radar reflector | | one |

*Note:* In some cases EPIRBs may not be part of the liferaft equipment, but will be carried on each side of the ship and stowed so they can be rapidly placed in any survival craft.

## Lifeboat equipment

| Item | Quantity |
|---|---|
| Oars | sufficient buoyant oars to make headway in calm seas |
| Crutches | one for each oar provided |
| Boat hooks | two |
| Plugs | two per plughole (except where automatic valves are fitted) |
| Buoyant bailer, buckets | one bailer and two rustproof buckets |
| Rudder and tiller | one each |
| Hatchets | two, one at each end of the lifeboat |
| Lamp | one with oil for 12 hours (older boats only) |
| Matches | two watertight containers |
| Mast and sail | one mast, with orange-coloured sails (Note: motor and mechanically propelled lifeboats are not required to carry mast and sails.) |
| Torch, waterproof, signalling | one, with a spare set of batteries and a spare bulb |
| Heliograph | one daylight signalling mirror |
| Knife | one, attached to boat by lanyard |
| Buoyant heaving lines | two, with rescue quoits attached |
| Whistle | one, or equivalent sound signal |
| Fishing kit | one, fishing line and six hooks |
| Exposure cover | one cover of a highly visible colour |
| Rescue signal table, used by life-saving stations, marine rescue units, ships and persons in distress | one copy |
| Lifeline | one, becketed around the outside |

| | |
|---|---|
| Small gear lockers | for stowage of small items of equipment |
| Painters | two painters: one secured to the forward end of the lifeboat with strop and toggle for quick release, the other secured to the stem of the lifeboat and ready for use |
| Seasickness tablets | six tablets per person |
| First aid outfit | one with instructions (see note) |
| Pump, manual, self-priming | one |
| Wave oil | 4.5 litres of animal, fish or vegetable oil with oil bag (older boats only) |
| Keel rails and grab lines | bilge keel rails, and grab lines secured from gunwale to gunwale under the keel (not required on self-righting boats) |
| Fire extinguishers (motor boats) | two, suitable for quenching oil fires |
| Survival instructions | one copy of *Survival at Sea* |
| Food ration | Food giving not less than 10,000 kilojoules for each person (667g per person) |
| Water ration | 3.0 litres of fresh water for each person the lifeboat is permitted to accommodate of which 1.0 litre per person may be replaced by a de-salting apparatus capable of producing 1 litre of fresh water in two days |
| Compass in a binnacle fitted with lamp | one |
| Sea anchor with hawser and tripping line | one |
| Parachute distress rockets, red | four |
| Hand flares, red | six |
| Buoyant smoke signals, orange | two |
| Tin openers | three |
| Searchlight | one, motor boats only |
| Efficient radar reflector | one |
| Thermal protective aid | sufficient for 10% of the boat's capacity or two, whichever is greater |
| Seasickness bag | one per person |
| Tools | sufficient tools for minor adjustmens to the engine and its accessories |

| | |
|---|---|
| Boarding ladder | one |
| A rust-proof dipper | one |
| A rust-proof graduated drinking vessel | one |

*Note:* New lifeboats have a manually controlled lamp fitted to the top of the cover, or enclosure, and a source of light inside the lifeboat.

*Note:* Narcotic drugs are normally kept in custody of the Master.

## Rescue boat equipment

Sufficient buoyant oars or paddles to make headway in calm seas

Thole pins or crutches for each oar

A buoyant bailer

A binnacle containing an efficient compass, which is luminous or has means of illumination

A sea anchor and tripping line, and hawser not less than 10m in length

A painter attached to a quick release device

A buoyant line not less than 50m in length for towing

A waterproof electric signalling torch, spare batteries and spare bulb

A whistle or equivalent sound signal

A first aid outfit in a waterproof case

Two buoyant rescue quoits; each attached to at least 30m of buoyant line

A searchlight

An efficient radar reflector

Thermal protective aids sufficient for 10% of the boat capacity or two, whichever is greater

Additional equipment for a rigid rescue boat:
i) a boat hook
ii) a bucket
iii) a knife or hatchet

Additional equipment for an inflated rescue boat:
i) a buoyant safety knife
ii) two sponges
iii) a bellows or pump
iv) a repair kit
v) a safety boat hook

*Note:* Rescue boats on pre-1986 ships may be equipped to lower standards.

## WATER AND FOOD

### Water

Water is essential for survival and is provided in all lifeboats, survival capsules and liferafts. Lifeboats and survival capsules carry 3.0 litres of fresh water for each person they are certified to carry, and liferafts carry 1. litres of fresh water for each person, the smaller mount being due to the restrictions on size and weight or packing into the rafts.

Survivors are faced with two problems in connection with drinking water: issuing the ration provided, and supplementing the ration.

## Issuing the water ration

There are two basic rules for survivors to follow when issuing the water ration:

No water should be issued in the first 24 hours in the survival craft (except to the sick and injured and in cases of excessive seasickness).

The normal ration per person per day is 0.5 a litre (500 millilitres).

When survivors abandon ship their bodies are full of water, therefore drinking water during the first 24 hours will result in the loss of water as urine. During the first 24 hours the body will become drier and better able to absorb the water ration on the second and subsequent days.

An exception is made for survivors who have been wounded or badly burned and who therefore have lost body fluids. They should start their water ration on the first day.

The daily ration of 500 ml is sufficient to sustain survivors providing they avoid dehydration and reduce sweating. It is important that this daily ration be issued. The temptation to cut down on the ration should be resisted as this will weaken survivors quickly and lessen the chance of survival.

It is recommended that the water ration be issued in three parts at sunrise, midday and sunset. At these times one-third of a day's ration (167 ml) should be issued to each survivor. The ration should be drunk slowly. Holding water in the mouth and gargling before swallowing helps to get the most value from the water.

Survivors should realise the difference between artificial thirst, as a result of thinking about water or of eating or drinking something containing salt, and real thirst. Real thirst means complete dryness of the mouth and throat with intense irritation.

On the last day of the water ration which will be the fourth day in a liferaft and the seventh day in a lifeboat providing no other water is obtained, the day's water ration should be halved to provide some water for the following day.

Where the drinking water has been supplemented by various means, the extra water should be issued first, and should be issued at the daily ration of 500 ml. The survival craft's water, and particularly the canned or packaged water in liferafts, should be kept as a reserve as it will keep in good condition for a longer period than rain water.

### Morale

It is important that every ration of water is properly measured in the sight of the recipient and of other survivors.

## Supplementing the water ration

All survivors should be aware of the importance of supplementing their drinking water by any available means. Although search and rescue facilities are designed for early location and rescue this may not always be possible, and survivors should think ahead beyond the duration of their water rations, particularly in liferafts where the water is only provided for the second, third, fourth and possibly the fifth day.

The drinking water ration can only be supplemented to any great extent by collecting rain water. It is therefore necessary for survivors to look out for approaching rain so that the occupants of survival craft are prepared to collect it, and so that powered craft can tow other craft into the path of passing rain showers.

In liferafts rain may be collected in the following manner:

- pull the drainage tube down and secure to depress canopy, and prepare containers, bags, etc.;
- wash off any salt encrustation with sea water just prior to rain commencing;
- fill every available empty container with rainwater, such as plastic bags, empty water tins, equipment bag, bowls, shoes and emergency pack; and
- if rainfall persists, drink your fill of water and use it for personal hygiene.

In lifeboats, which have a larger initial water capacity, survivors should use whatever methods are available. In particular, a flexible exposure cover might be used as a rainwater catchment by piercing one or two holes and by securing a rope to pull it down. Any water 'caught' can drain into buckets and bags such as the exposure cover bag and the sea anchor bag. Small containers such as those used for pyrotechnics and small items of equipment are also handy for storing rainwater.

It is also likely that water will condense on the inner lining of liferaft canopies and on the inside of lifeboat covers. This water should be collected with sponges or cloths used only for that purpose and therefore not contaminated with sea water or other matter.

## Food

Food is not essential for survival over a short period of time. However, a limited food ration is supplied to assist the water economy of the body, to provide energy enabling work to be done, and to aid morale.

The food provided in survival craft consists of barley sugar or proprietary brands of long-life food in accordance with international requirements.

It is important to understand that the food provided in survival craft is chosen on the basis of the water used in its breakdown in the body. Proteins and fats require ample water for complete digestion, whereas carbohydrates, such as barley sugar, will help to conserve water in the body. A ration closely approaching 100% carbohydrate is therefore most suitable for long-term survival in a survival craft.

The total food ration provided is 10,000 kilojoules for each person that a lifeboat or liferaft is permitted to accommodate.

### Issuing the food ration

The following rules should be followed when issuing the food ration:

- No food should be issued in the first 24 hours (except for the sick and injured) as the body's needs can be met from previous meals.
- The daily ration per person in survival craft after the first day should total 165 grams in lifeboats and 125 grams in liferafts. Since each 'sweet' is 5 grams this means 33 or 25 pieces of barley sugar per day for each person.
- The food should be issued once or twice a day.

It may not be possible to divide the food exactly into the correct proportions. It is suggested that one tin, packet, jar, etc, be opened at a time, and the contents counted out in the sight of the recipients.

### Morale

It is extremely important for morale that the issue of food and water is fair and this is seen to be so by others in the survival craft.

### Supplementing the food ration

Survivors must realise that hunger in itself is not harmful, especially over short periods, and that providing adequate drinking water is available it is possible to survive for as long as seven to eight weeks without food. Supplementing the food ration, although desirable, is not a necessity.

If the ration is to be supplemented while at sea in survival craft (survival on land is discussed later) the sources of additional food are limited. If and when caught the eating of such foods should depend upon the availability of additional drinking water.

Possible sources of additional food, depending upon position and sea temperature, are: fish, birds, seaweed, plankton, and turtles.

### Fish

The most likely source of additional food is fish, especially as a basic fishing tackle is provided in the survival craft. Survivors should also be alert for the possibility of flying fish landing in the survival craft.

Most fish caught in the open sea are likely to be edible, but survivors should be aware of the various dangerous types of fish that have spines, spikes or bristles or that puff themselves up. These should not be touched as their spines or flesh may contain strong poisons for which no antidote is available in survival craft. Cases are known of such venom causing death.

When catching fish, survivors should attempt to catch only small fish and try to avoid losing the line or hooks. If necessary improvised fish hooks and lines can be made from small items. The fishing line should not be secured to the craft or around the body. It is best to have other survivors holding the inboard end of the line.

There are two ways of using any fish that may be caught. The water in the fish may be obtained by chewing the flesh and spitting out the residue, or the flesh can be cut into thin strips up to 2 cm thick and dried in the sun for eating later.

Remember that additional drinking water must be available for consumption when eating or sucking fish. Fish should preferably be dried and kept until heavy rainfall.

Survivors should also consider using materials in the survival craft to fashion a spear or gaff for catching fish.

Do not fish if sharks are near. Abandon a fish if a shark appears, even with the loss of line and hook.

### Birds

All sea birds, except albatrosses, are edible although the taste may not be attractive to survivors. Birds can be caught with fish skin or other bait wrapped around a strong hook.

### Seaweed

Seaweeds are more likely to be found in coastal water but may also be found in deeper waters due to

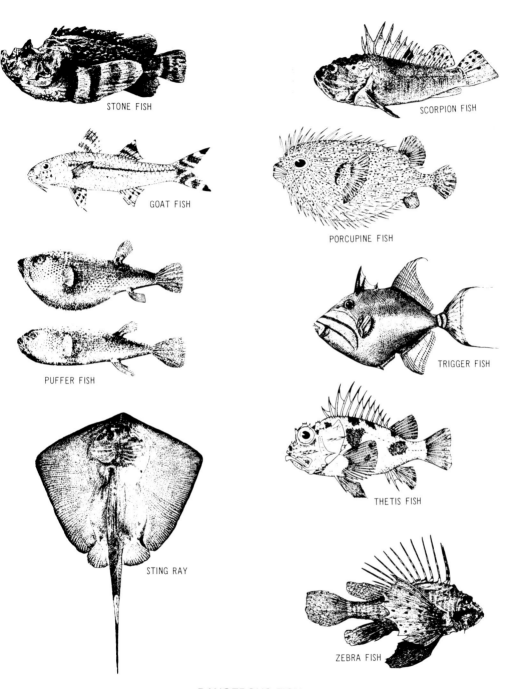

STONE FISH

SCORPION FISH

GOAT FISH

PORCUPINE FISH

PUFFER FISH

TRIGGER FISH

STING RAY

THETIS FISH

ZEBRA FISH

DANGEROUS FISH

currents. Most seaweeds are edible and resemble green vegetables but, because they are salty, should be eaten only when additional water is available. Seaweeds should be carefully inspected for small shellfish and organisms before eating as these may be poisonous.

### Plankton

This consists of minute animals and plants which are consumed by fish. Plankton is suitable as a food and is tasty in small amounts, but because it is very salty should be eaten only when additional drinking water is available. Small quantities of plankton may be obtained by dragging a net of very fine material behind a moving survival craft.

### Turtles

In waters they frequent, turtles offer a major source of food if they can be caught. It is recommended that only survivors in lifeboats attempt to catch them, as the beak or the claws on the flippers could damage liferafts.

The turtle should be pulled into the boat, turned on its back, killed by cutting its throat with the lifeboat axe and the belly shell removed. The blood is a valuable source of nourishment and should be drunk before it coagulates. The keeping quality of the meat will be improved if the turtle is bled.

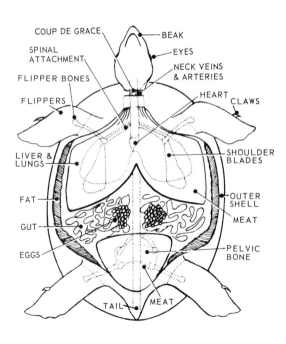

TURTLE — FOOD PARTS

Not only does the turtle provide a supply of meat which can be dried and kept for later eating, but female turtles may contain a large number of eggs, which can be mixed with the normal emergency rations.

The green turtle is preferred for food; studies indicate the hawksbill turtle may be dangerous.

### Basic points when supplementing the food ration

If other food can be obtained, survivors must remember three basic points:

- Eating food other than pure carbohydrates (such as barley sugar), and especially salty foods, requires more drinking water than the normal daily ration provides.
- Extra food, or parts of fishes, birds, etc, thought to be unsuitable for consumption must be left well alone. All extra food should first be carefully tasted.
- Offal should not be dumped in the sea when sharks are present because of possible damage to liferaft or boats by frenzied sharks.

### LOOKOUT

The lookout is the eyes and ears for the occupants of survival craft. While most tasks performed by survivors are carried out inside the survival craft, the lookout duty is concerned with things outside the craft. In most cases the lookout is cut off from the rest of the survivors and exposed to the weather outside the shelter of the survival craft.

Lookout duties must therefore be shared between the survivors so that the time on watch takes account of outside conditions and the risks of exposure, sunburn etc. It is preferable that a lookout is posted for 24 hours a day.

The lookout's duties consist of keeping continuous all-round watch for:

### Rainshowers

Because of the need to supplement the drinking water rations, no opportunity for collecting rainwater should be neglected. It is necessary to see in good time any approaching clouds likely to bring rain so that other survivors can prepare for collecting the rainwater. Clouds likely to bring rain are either layer clouds of middle and low altitude which will ususaly give continuous rain or clouds of great vertical height which will give showers of rain or hail. Containers for rainwater should be kept clean and free of any salt or other contamination.

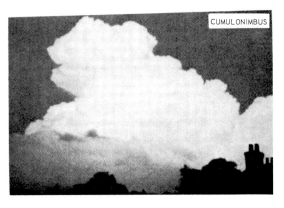

CUMULONIMBUS

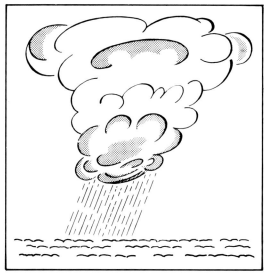

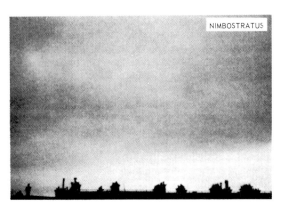

NIMBOSTRATUS

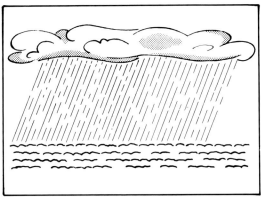

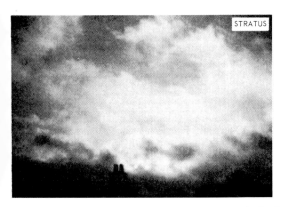

STRATUS

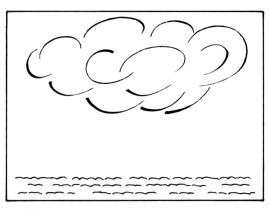

CLOUD TYPES

43

## Food sources

Lookouts should watch for the approach of possible sources for supplementing the food ration, i.e. fish, birds, turtles, seaweed.

## Indications of land

In addition to the possibility of sighting lights or land, lookouts should know the following indications of land:

### Certain cloud types

Some varieties of cloud are formed over land due to the faster heating of land compared with sea, or due to high ground. Cumulus cloud may form over land masses during the morning and dissipate at night. Small cumulus clouds may form over islands and then move downwind when there are no other cloud systems. Clouds that appear not to move and are of flattened cumulus type may be formed over hills or mountains.

### Smoke

Smoke coming from a stationary source or a steady direction may be from industrial sources on land or from bushfires.

### Loom or glare from lights

The lights from small towns beneath the horizon might give rise to a steady glow in the sky at night.

Similarly, an intermittent glow may be the loom of a light from a lighthouse or aircraft beacon.

### Sea-birds

Most varieties of sea-birds return to the coast each night and rarely travel more than 100 miles out to sea. In the morning sea-birds may be seen flying away from land, in the early evening returning to land.

### Outflow from rivers

The outflow from rivers, especially in the rainy season, may cause areas of discoloured water with sharply defined demarcation between fresh and salt water. Such outflows may also be indicated by logs and vegetation carried out to sea. In addition, the fresh water may have a noticeable sickly smell.

### Coral reefs

With out-lying low coral reefs the indications are likely to be a sickly smell, the sound of breakers, a green tint to the sky or the under side of clouds from sunlight reflected from shallow lagoons, and a luminous glow from breakers at night.

### Land and sea breezes

These can be noticed by the reversal of the wind direction, the dominant breeze being towards the land from mid-morning to evening, and from the land at night.

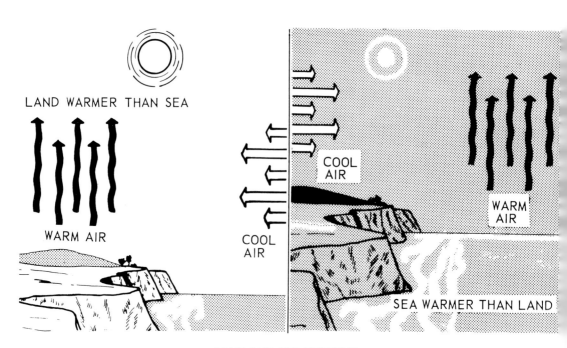

LAND WARMER THAN SEA

WARM AIR

COOL AIR

COOL AIR

WARM AIR

SEA WARMER THAN LAND

**LAND AND SEA BREEZES**

# Ships

Lookouts should always watch for approaching ships or small craft by day or night. Although the visual horizon from a lifeboat or liferaft may only be two miles, the masts or lights of a ship that is 'hull down' will be seen much further away. Lookouts should watch for masts, mastlights, funnels, smoke, and sun reflecting from the superstructure of ships.

Attempt to attract the attention of any ships sighted by the means detailed in Chapter 5.

# Aircraft

Lookouts should watch for aircraft passing over or near the survival craft. Aircraft at a considerable height may be able to pick up signals from an EPIRB even when they are unable to sight survival craft.

Searching aircraft are likely to be flying at low or medium altitude following various search patterns; they may be heard before being seen.

Attempt to attract the attention of any aircraft sighted by the means detailed in Chapter 5.

# Dangers

Lookouts should also keep a watch for the approach of dangers to the survival craft, or the approach of the craft to dangers such as sharks and other voracious fish, stinging jellyfish, whales, squalls, breaking wave systems, rocks or reefs, and breakers.

Lookouts should report anything they see to the person in charge of the survival craft before taking any other action. In addition to the dangers mentioned above, lookouts should note all changing circumstances such as changes in wind direction, changes in sea or swell, changing types and amounts of cloud and cloud cover, and changing temperature.

# NAVIGATION

Although survival craft are recommended to stay as close as possible to the 'abandon ship' position except for possibly making for the coast, if near by, it may assist morale to work out their likely movement and position.

This knowledge is also useful if contact can be made with ships or with a coast radio station using the portable radio equipment, particularly if land is in sight and its direction can be found.

The simple navigation measures available to survivors include finding N-S or E-W directions, finding the direction of current and wind, and plotting an estimated position providing the actual or approximate 'abandon ship' position is known and the rate of drift can be estimated.

# Finding direction

There are four simple measures available:

## Direction of sun at noon

Remember that the sun rises in the east and sets in the west. If south of 23.5° south latitude, the sun will pass to the north of you and its highest altitude will indicate the direction of true north.

If north of 23.5° north latitude, the sun will pass to the south of you and will indicate south by its highest altitude. Between those two latitudes, in the tropics, the sun's path will be to the south or north depending on the latitude and the time of the year.

## Bearing of sunrise

The following table gives a guide to the true bearing of the sun at sunrise, according to the time of the year and the latitude. For dates and latitudes in between those shown, interpolate between the given bearings.

BEARING OF THE SUN AT TRUE SUNRISE
(i.e. when lower limb of sun is half of sun's diameter above the horizon)

| Latitude | 5 Feb. | 20 March | 6 May | 21 June |
|---|---|---|---|---|
| 60°N | 124° | 090° | 056° | 037° |
| 45°N | 113° | 090° | 067° | 055° |
| 30°N | 109° | 090° | 071° | 063° |
| 15°N | 107° | 090° | 073° | 065° |
| 0° | 106° | 090° | 074° | 067° |
| 15°S | 107° | 090° | 073° | 065° |
| 30°S | 109° | 090° | 071° | 063° |
| 45°S | 113° | 090° | 067° | 055° |
| Latitude | 7 Aug. | 22 Sept. | 6 Nov. | 21 Dec. |
| 60°N | 056° | 090° | 124° | 143° |
| 45°N | 067° | 090° | 113° | 125° |
| 30°N | 071° | 090° | 109° | 117° |
| 15°N | 073° | 090° | 107° | 115° |
| 0° | 074° | 090° | 106° | 113° |
| 15°S | 073° | 090° | 107° | 115° |
| 30°S | 071° | 090° | 109° | 117° |
| 45°S | 067° | 090° | 113° | 125° |

The sun's bearing at true sunset can be obtained by subtracting the tabled bearings from 360°.

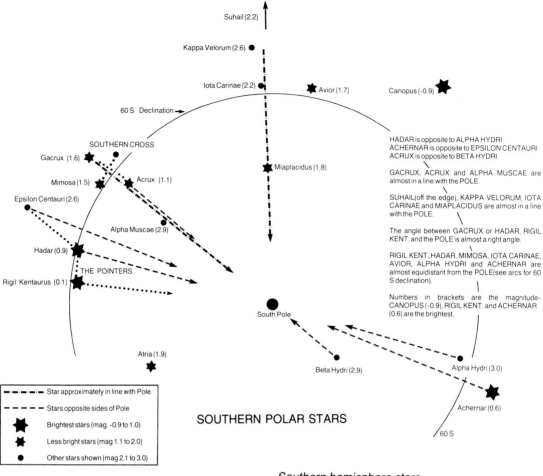

Suhail (2.2)

Kappa Velorum (2.6) ●

Iota Carinae (2.2) ●          Avior (1.7)          Canopus (-0.9)

60 S Declination →

SOUTHERN CROSS
Gacrux (1.6)          Miaplacidus (1.8)
Mimosa (1.5)     Acrux (1.1)
Epsilon Centauri (2.6)
Alpha Muscae (2.9)
Hadar (0.9)
THE POINTERS
Rigil Kentaurus (0.1)

South Pole

Atria (1.9)

Beta Hydri (2.9)          Alpha Hydri (3.0)

Achernar (0.6)

60 S

HADAR is opposite to ALPHA HYDRI
ACHERNAR is opposite to EPSILON CENTAURI
ACRUX is opposite to BETA HYDRI

GACRUX, ACRUX and ALPHA MUSCAE are almost in a line with the POLE.

SUHAIL(off the edge), KAPPA VELORUM, IOTA CARINAE and MIAPLACIDUS are almost in a line with the POLE.

The angle between GACRUX or HADAR, RIGIL KENT. and the POLE is almost a right angle.

RIGIL KENT.,HADAR, MIMOSA, IOTA CARINAE, AVIOR, ALPHA HYDRI and ACHERNAR are almost equidistant from the POLE(see arcs for 60 S declination).

Numbers in brackets are the magnitude- CANOPUS (-0.9), RIGIL KENT. and ACHERNAR (0.6) are the brightest.

—·—·—·— Star approximately in line with Pole

— — — — Stars opposite sides of Pole

★ Brightest stars (mag. -0.9 to 1.0)

✦ Less bright stars (mag 1.1 to 2.0)

● Other stars shown (mag 2.1 to 3.0)

### SOUTHERN POLAR STARS

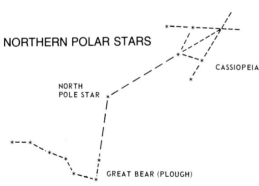

### NORTHERN POLAR STARS

CASSIOPEIA

NORTH
POLE STAR

GREAT BEAR (PLOUGH)

### Northern hemisphere stars

The Pole Star stays almost right above the North Pole and, if visible, gives a good indication of the N. direction. To find the Pole Star, survivors can use the constellations of the Great Bear (Plough) or Cassiopeia as shown.

Note that Cassiopeia and the Plough are on opposite sides of the Pole Star.

### Southern hemisphere stars

An indication of the direction of true south can be obtained from the Southern Cross, from part of Centaurus, and from Achernar, as shown.

### Estimating the rate of downwind movement

Providing that the average wind velocity can be obtained by reference to the sea state using the Beaufort Scale, this rate is easy to estimate.

For inflatable liferafts the rate is about six per cent of the average wind velocity when the drogue is not streamed, and about three per cent of average wind velocity when the drogue is streamed. Rigid liferafts could be expected to move downwind at a slightly slower rate due to the ballast and drag of the water trapped by the lower canopy.

It can be assumed that liferafts will always go downwind, but they may drift up to 60° either side o. the direct downwind direction.

The graph on page 34 indicates the rates of downwind movement for inflatable liferafts.

## BEAUFORT WIND SCALE
(for an effective height of 10 metres
above sea level)

| Beaufort Number | Descriptive Term | Wind Speed knots | Deep Sea Criterion | Wave Height metres |
|---|---|---|---|---|
| 0 | Calm | <1 | Sea like a mirror | |
| 1 | Light air | 1-3 | Ripples with the appearance of scales are formed, but without foam crests | 0.1 |
| 2 | Light breeze | 4-6 | Small wavelets, still short but more pronounced; crests have a glassy appearance and do not break | 0.2 |
| 3 | Gentle breeze | 7-10 | Large wavelets; crests begin to break; foam of glassy appearance; perhaps scattered white horses | 0.6 |
| 4 | Moderate breeze | 11-16 | Small waves, becoming longer; fairly frequent white horses | 1 |
| 5 | Fresh breeze | 17-21 | Moderate waves, taking a more pronounced long form; many white horses are formed (chance of some spray) | 2 |
| 6 | Strong breeze | 22-27 | Large waves begin to form; the white foam crests are more extensive everywhere (probably some spray) | 3 |
| 7 | Near gale | 28-33 | Sea heaps up and white foam from breaking waves begins to be blown in streaks along the direction of the wind | 4 |
| 8 | Gale | 34-40 | Moderately high waves of greater length; edges of crests begin to break into spindrift; foam is blown in well-marked streaks along the direction of the wind | 5.5 |
| 9 | Strong gale | 41-47 | High waves; dense streaks of foam along the direction of the wind; crests of waves begin to topple, rumble and roll over; spray may affect visibility | 7 |
| 10 | Storm | 48-55 | Very high waves with long overhanging crests; the resulting foam, in great patches, is blown in dense white streaks along the direction of the wind; on the whole, the surface of the sea takes a white appearance; the tumbling of the sea becomes heavy and shock-like; visibility affected | 9 |
| 11 | Violent storm | 56-63 | Exceptionally high waves (small and medium-sized ships might be for a time lost to view behind the waves); the sea is completely covered with long white patches of foam lying along the direction of the wind; everywhere the edges of the wave crests are blown into froth; visibility affected | 11.5 |
| 12 | Hurricane | 64 and over | The air is filled with foam and spray; sea completely white with driving spray; visibility very seriously affected | 14 |

For lifeboats, the rates are slightly less than those of liferafts, being five per cent of average wind velocity when the sea anchor is not streamed, and two and a half per cent when it is streamed. Lifeboats are likely to move up to 40° either side of the downwind direction.

## Estimated position

For survivors estimating their position after moving downwind in survival craft it is necessary to know the abandon ship position, direction(s) of wind, period of time moving downwind in each direction, and rate(s) of downwind movement for each period. It is then possible to find the distance in each direction, and to make a simple plot or diagram to find the position to which the craft has moved under the influence of the wind.

One other factor must be considered — current. Away from the coast, currents are likely to be slow and steady, while in coastal waters tidal currents will vary in set and rate.

The rate of ocean currents is generally one to two knots or less but in certain areas the rate may increase to two to three knots or higher. Such rates are found in the major current systems of the North and South Pacific and Atlantic Oceans and in the Indian Ocean. In many parts of the oceans currents are so variable that no general set can be discerned. (See Charts of Ocean Currents and Sea Surface Currents in Australian Waters in Appendix C.)

Survivors should also be aware that current systems often contain large eddies which produce an apparent fluctuation in strength and direction. This is most marked when currents and eddies impinge on coastlines or the edge of the continental shelf, for example, the East Australian Coast Current. Inshore of the main stream a reverse set is often found, and this may be very marked close inshore, especially if the shoreline consists of headlands and bays.

To find an estimated position, apply the set and drift of the current to the position found from the effect of the wind.

Remember that any information on positions or bearings which survivors can pass on by means of radio can be of vital importance in bringing about their rescue. In particular, if survivors can advise a radio station of the extact instant of sunrise or sunset it will be possible for the SAR authority to calculate a position line to assist in the search.

# Chapter 4
# Medical Duties

This chapter covers the treatment of survivors injured before or during abandonment, for whom first aid needs to be continued. It also covers the care of survivors in the survival craft.

Wherever possible, the person in charge of a survival craft, or of a group of survival craft, should nominate a survivor skilled in first aid to take charge of medical duties. Such a person would preferably have completed a course of first aid training.

It is useful to group injured persons together, as far as possible, taking account of the nature of their injuries and the possible dangers of moving them.

Where survival craft are separated or where no survivor has first aid training, the leader of each craft should nominate a fit survivor to carry out their duties according to these instructions, using the first aid kit common to all survival craft.

## CONTENTS OF THIS CHAPTER
**Medical duties**
> Contents and use of the first aid kit
> The signs of death
> Treating survivors injured before or during
> abandonment
> Treating the apparently drowned and asphyxiated
> Treating unconsciousness
> Treating shock
> Treating wounds
> Treating burns
> Treating fractures
> Treating oil fuel contamination

**Long-term care for survivors**
> Hypothermia
> Immersion foot
> Frostbite
> Sunburn
> Salt water boils and sores
> Body functions
> Dehydration
> Delirium and mental disturbance
> Hygiene

## MEDICAL DUTIES
### Contents and use of the first aid kit

Morphine sulphate injections — five doses, or
Pentazocine injections — five doses, or
Omnopon Tubunic — six doses

One pack is provided containing either five or six doses of these injections, which are used for relieving severe pain from burns, wound, fractures and other causes. A second injection may be made in half an hour if necessary, but the patient should not have a third injection until six hours later, and then only if still restless or in pain. The dose for adults is not more than three injections in 24 hours.

Records must be kept of time and amount of these injections.

*Note:* These injections will normally be kept in the custody of the ship's Master. They must be brought to the survival craft before abandonment.

*Standard dressings*

Eight are provided, in two sizes. They consist of a pad of sterilised gauze attached to a bandage. These are used to dress large wounds with the pad being placed directly over the wound.

*Triangular bandages*

Six are provided. These can be used as slings or for bandaging purposes.

*Open weave bandages*

Ten bandages, each 5 metres in length, are provided for dressing small wounds or for securing burn dressings or splints.

*Waterproof self-adhesive dressings*

One packet of assorted size dressings for small wounds.

*Paraffin gauze dressings*

One packet containing 10 individually wrapped dressings is provided. These are used for dressing burns according to the instructions on the packet.

*Cetrimide cream*

Two tubes of this antiseptic cream are provided. Apply to contaminated or infected wounds or burns after cleaning the burn with cool water (if possible) and for septic skin conditions such as boils.

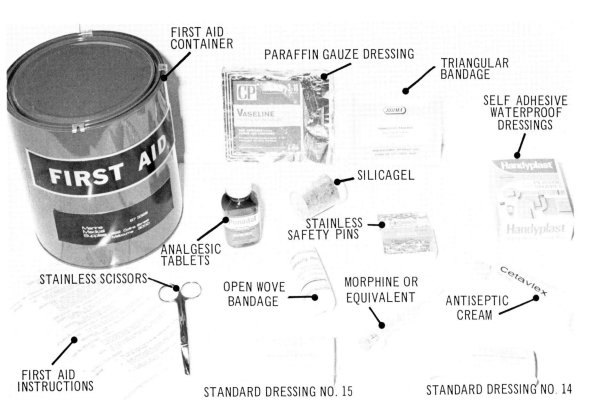

FIRST AID CONTAINER — PARAFFIN GAUZE DRESSING — TRIANGULAR BANDAGE — SELF ADHESIVE WATERPROOF DRESSINGS — SILICAGEL — STAINLESS SAFETY PINS — ANALGESIC TABLETS — STAINLESS SCISSORS — OPEN WOVE BANDAGE — MORPHINE OR EQUIVALENT — ANTISEPTIC CREAM — FIRST AID INSTRUCTIONS — STANDARD DRESSING NO. 15 — STANDARD DRESSING NO. 14

FIRST AID CONTAINER AND CONTENTS

*Paracetamol tablets (similar use as aspirin or codeine)*

These are used to relieve pain of any kind not serious enough for the use of morphine. Dose is two tablets, repeated three to four times per day.

*Scissors*

For cutting and trimming bandages, etc. and for cutting away clothing where necessary. Do not use for any other purpose.

*Instructions for use of first aid kit*

Approved instructions are included.

*Recommendations:*

The following items which are not included in the first aid kit are recommended as optional:
  (a) Betadine (a povidone iodine solution)
  (b) Sunscreen 15+; or Ungvita containing vitamin A; a superficial burn cream may be used
  (c) Friar's Balsam

**The signs of death**

In treating survivors, it also necessary to know how to recognise the death of badly injured or drowned persons. Signs which should be used as a guide are given in Appendix A, together with comments on the burial of the dead.

> **WARNING: severe hypothermia resembles death!**

**Treating survivors injured before or during abandonment**

Give first aid in accordance with the instructions in the first aid kit, or standard first aid practice.

**Treating the apparently drowned and asphyxiated**

Asphyxia is a condition caused by a breakdown in the supply of oxygen to the body resulting from a failure of the respiratory system due to:

49

- the obstruction of chest movements, i.e. from injury;
- insufficient or obstructed supply of oxygen;
- effects of poisoning, shock, heart failure.

Survivors from a life-saving incident are most likely to be asphyxiated due to chest injuries or obstruction of air passages (particularly due to intake of water), and shock.

Unless the cause of asphyxia can be quickly removed and the supply of oxygen restored there is:

- cessation of breathing;
- loss of consciousness;
- failure of circulation.

The signs of asphyxia are:

- changes in rate and depth of breathing;
- cyanosis of face, lips, ears and nail beds of fingers and toes (they turn blue);
- the veins of neck and head are swollen;
- the blood vessels of the eyes are swollen and red;
- gasping respiration;
- noisy breathing with frothing may develop;
- consciousness is lost;
- fits may occur;
- breathing may stop;
- the heart may stop.

Treating asphyxiated survivors consists of four steps:

- separate the patient from the cause of asphyxia, e.g. take out of water;
- ensure a clear airway;
- restore the circulation, if necessary;
- restore breathing.

A clear airway is ensured by laying the patient on his or her back, pressing the top of the head downwards with a backward tilt of the head and lifting the jaw forward with a pistol type grip; this will help to clear the tongue from the airway. Remove any food, mucus or other matter from the mouth. When opening and clearing the airway, the casualty should not be supine as something in the mouth could fall back and block the airway. It is good practice to roll the casualty onto his or her side to clear and open the airway, then if there is no breathing, the casualty is rolled onto the back for expired air resuscitation (EAR).

*Note:* the tongue is the most common cause of airway obstruction — it can fall back and block the windpipe in an unconscious casualty.

If necessary, and if the patient is not suffering from chest injuries, circulation can sometimes be restored by external cardiac compression. This is carried out by putting intermittent pressure on the lower chest to compress the heart between the lower part of the breast bone and the spinal column to simulate the normal contraction of the heart. Pressure is applied using the heel of each hand, one above the other and repeated. External cardiac compression should be combined with the mouth to mouth method of artificial respiration (CPR). The following rates are recommended:

Adults: 1 Person CPR — press at a rate of 70–80 per minute. Give two breaths after each 15 compressions (4 cycles/minute), delivering 60 compressions/minute to the heart.

2 Person CPR — 1 breath every 5 compressions, preferably without pausing with compression while breath is applied. Apply 12 cycles/minute.

*Note:* Depth of compression for adults should be 4–5 cms.

Extreme care should be taken when dealing with children/babies, where the rate of compression is faster, but the compression depth lower.

### Mouth to mouth resuscitation

With this method exhaled air is forced into the lungs of a survivor whose breathing has stopped or is failing.

With the patient on his or her back, and with a clear airway obtained, kneel beside the head, and:

- supporting jaw with pistol grip, open patient's mouth;
- seal lips around the patient's mouth, or mouth and nose for a baby;
- pinch patient's nostrils between thumb and forefinger;
- breathe out firmly into patient's mouth and watch the chest rise as in normal respiration;
- remove mouth;
- allow patient's chest to collapse.

Give five quick breaths, then check pulse. If there is a pulse, continue expired air resuscitation (EAR) at 4–5 second intervals. If there is no pulse, commence mouth to mouth resuscitation together with chest compressions.

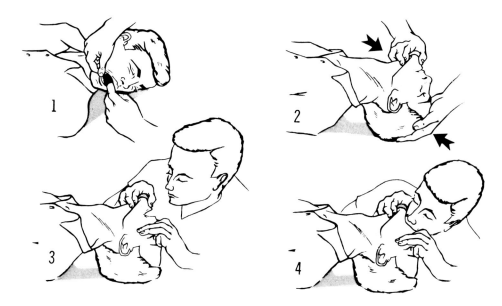

MOUTH TO MOUTH RESUSCITATION

### Mouth to nose method

Where the patient's mouth is injured or blocked, inflation of the chest can be achieved by putting the first aider's mouth to the patient's nose.

The method is similar to the mouth to mouth method. The patient's mouth does not need to be open for air expirations, unless there is some reason the air cannot escape through the nose.

Important points with these methods:

Air must enter and leave the patient's lungs.

The chest must rise and fall.

The patient's head must be correctly placed throughout.

An airtight seal must be be maintained during exhalation into the patient's mouth or nose.

The operator should watch for a collapse of chest and should take in fresh air for the next inflation.

When patient commences to breathe, continue assisting the breathing, and watching rise and fall of the patient's chest to attempt to keep in step with the attempts to breathe.

Put the patient on his or her side when breathing is established.

Artificial respiration should be continued for at least four hours if the patient shows no signs of recovery, unless the person in charge is satisfied that the signs of death are present. To carry out artificial respiration for such a period of time in a survival craft is very demanding and it is likely that a team of two or three operators will be required to carry out the task.

### Treating unconsciousness

Unconsciousness may appear either as a retarding of mental activity or as a deeply comatose state. Unconsciousness can be progressive and regular re-examination of the patient is necessary. The patient may be in danger from an inability to react to or appreciate danger, inability to maintain a clear airway, and from inadequate circulation or respiration. Treatment consists of these steps:

- Clear obstruction to airway.
- Check pulse. If absent, commence external cardiac compression to stimulate circulation.
- Check breathing. If stopped or weak, commence artificial respiration.
- Control any bleeding.
- Check for any other injuries, particularly to the spine.
- Place patient in the coma position.

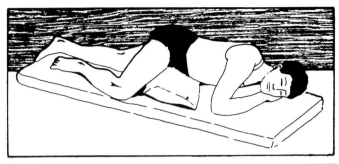

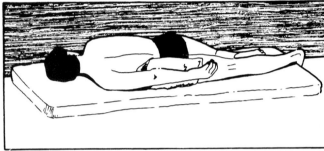

COMA POSITION

- Assess the level of consciousness by the response to touch, command or pain, the state of breathing, the size and reaction of pupils — normal pupils are equal in size and react to light by getting smaller — and by whether patient is quiet or restless.
- Loosen clothing around neck, chest and waist.
- Watch colour of patient. If patient's colour has not paled, circulation is adequate.
- Do not give anything by mouth.

The causes of unconsciousness are many — head injuries, fits, heart attacks, drunkenness, asphyxia, poisons or shock — and the signs of unconsciousness vary accordingly.

The coma position is a position in which unconscious patients are placed so that secretions, blood, vomit, food, etc. may drain from the mouth and not obstruct the airway. It is a position for patients whose circulation and respiration are satisfactory or who are recovering.

To place the patient in the coma position in a survival craft will require the use of as large an area of flat space as possible, and the cooperation of the other occupants. If the patient is lying on the back:

- cross patient's right leg over left leg;
- kneel at patient's side;
- place patient's right arm across his or her chest;
- put left arm flat alongside body, palm up; tuck hand under buttock (at 45° angle), the lower shoulder will not go behind to stabilise the position;
- roll patient onto left side;
- bend patient's right leg up to a right angle and if necessary support it with something;
- place the patient's right hand under left cheek;
- turn the head to one side in a backward tilted position;
- gently pull patient's shoulder through to the back to maintain the position.

**Treating shock**

Shock is a state of collapse caused by a reduction in the volume of blood circulating in the body due to loss of blood, serum or fluids.

Shock may be caused by severe bleeding, burns, injuries, disease and infections, poisons, heart attacks, heat exhaustion, or due to a nervous reaction after injury or a severe fright.

Shock develops when the heart beats faster as it attempts to maintain normal blood pressure and the pulse becomes rapid and feeble. The brain receives less oxygen due to the low blood pressure and decreased volume of blood circulating, and dizziness, fainting and unconsciousness can occur.

Survivors affected by shock are likely to have a cold, clammy skin, a slow pulse that becomes rapid and feeble, shallow and rapid respiration, and may show early or later signs of unconsciousness. In addition, they may be affected by giddiness and fainting, thirst, nausea and vomiting.

Treatment consists of these steps:

- Ensure clear airway and adequate ventilation.
- Control any bleeding.
- Place an unconscious patient in coma position.
- If conscious ensure maximum supply of blood to the brain by placing patient on back and raising legs.
- Prevent patient from shivering, without warming the patient too much.

  Relieve pain by treatment of injuries.
- Reassure and encourage the patient.
- Do not give sips of water if patient is unconscious, unable to swallow, has an abdominal injury, or if the patient feels sick.

## Treating wounds

Wounds are cuts or tears in the body tissue which result in bleeding. When treating wounds it is necessary to stop the bleeding, to stop or prevent infection, prevent pain and reassure the patient.

### Bleeding

Bleeding is usually stopped in wounds by the natural formation of blood clots. Severe bleeding must be stopped as soon as possible:

Lay the patient flat and, if possible, raise the wounded part.

Expose the wound, cutting away clothing if necessary, but do not remove any blood clots.

Apply a standard dressing to the wound, folded to the correct size. Do not touch the part of dressing to be in contact with the wound.

Press the dressing firmly on; if blood soaks through, add more padding but do not remove dressing. Do not bandage until bleeding stops — keep up pressure with hand.

- Watch patient to make sure that bleeding has stopped. If it has not, apply more pressure.
- If there is very severe pain inject morphine, or give two paracetamol tablets for a lower level of pain.

Almost all cases of bleeding from wounds can be stopped by this method of applying pressure to dressings over the wound. In more severe cases, pressure over the artery bringing blood to the wound may also be required. This requires one person to put pressure over the artery and one person to apply a dressing to the wound as above. After 15 minutes, release pressure slowly to see if bleeding has stopped. Pressure over the artery should not need to be maintained for more than an hour.

A tourniquet can be used as a last resort for amputations where the limb is already lost, or for crater wounds (e.g. shark bite) where no other method will stop the bleeding. In these cases, however, there is often not much bleeding, because the wound is so massive that the surrounding muscles clamp and contract hard, thus effectively stopping the blood flow.

*Note*: Pressure over an artery should be applied by hand; a constrictive (i.e. wide) bandage should not be used.

### Preventing infection

Where a wound is contaminated, it should be cleaned before applying a dressing. Do not remove deeply impaled objects — bandage around them. The ends of long protruding objects, (e.g. fish spear) may be carefully cut off if necessary, but pulling the object out may cause more damage, especially if the object is plugging a torn organ or blood vessel. Unless the likelihood of rescue could be delayed, it is better to leave impaled objects in, for removal under correct medical supervision.

During bandaging or dressing of wounds, try not to touch surfaces which will be in contact with the wound, and try not to cough, sneeze, talk or breathe out directly towards the wound.

With small wounds the antiseptic cream can be applied immediately. With large wounds and severe bleeding, first control the bleeding, and keep the initial dressing on for a day or so. Then apply antiseptic cream to the healing wound and to any surrounding inflamed areas when re-dressing the wound.

## Treating burns

Burns are damage to body tissues caused by exposure of the tissues to excess heat or cold, which may be 'dry' heat, e.g. fire, flame, sunburn or contact with a hot object, 'moist' heat from hot water or steam, or cold from touching metallic objects in sub-zero air temperatures. All burns provide raw tissues susceptible to infection.

Burns are classified according to their depth, and to the area of the body surface burnt. Superficial burns are those where only the outer layers of skin are damaged; the area is red and painful and blisters may form. Deep burns are those where the full thickness of the skin is destroyed, and the underlying fat and muscle are burned; the area has a yellowish white or charred appearance.

The larger the area of the body burned, the greater the shock and the more seriously ill the patient. The chances of survival are related to the extent of burns on the body and not to their depth. All burns are serious, but burns exceeding 10 per cent of body surface are dangerous, and those exceeding 33 per cent are often fatal.

Shock occurs in burns because of loss of fluid from the blood, nervous reaction, which may be extreme, or pain. Infection can result in shock.

### Treating superficial burns

Cool with cold water for 10 minutes and cover with a sterile non-stick dressing. It is recommended that a paraffin gauze dressing should not be put on the wound until it starts to debride, possibly the following day. A dressing is not required if the skin is just red, not broken.

Survivors may be liable to prolonged exposure to the sun, which may lead to extensive superficial burns with formation of blisters. Serious sunburn with blistering should be treated with paraffin gauze dressings or with clean dry dressings and antiseptic cream. A sunscreen is recommended for the prevention and treatment of sunburn and other superficial burns.

### Treating deep burns

It is recommended that clothing stuck to a burn is not touched; trying to remove it could pull off further tissue, making the burn worse. Soaking the clothing may loosen stuck clothing, but some types which have melted (e.g. nylon) can be very hard to remove without tearing the tissue.

*Note*: Burns should only be treated if rescue is considered to be days away rather than hours; then treatment should take place after 24 hours. A light non-stick dressing can be used.

- Cool thoroughly (except old burns which can be washed, to remove debris).
- Cover burned area with paraffin gauze dressing, then apply a clean dressing and bandage securely.
- If burned area is extensive, cover with clean dressing over antiseptic solution and bandage firmly in position (see note above).
- Treat for pain and shock, giving morphine injection where necessary.
- Loosen bandages if swelling occurs.

Paraffin gauze dressings should be renewed daily until blistering has stopped. Then apply antiseptic cream and clean dressings.

## Treating fractures

A fracture is a broken bone, which may be the result of force applied to the bone, i.e. impact, force applied to an associated or linked bone, i.e. as in falling on the arms, or as a result of abnormal muscle action. Fractures are of three types:

- closed: where skin around fracture is unbroken;
- open: where a wound leads into the fracture, or the bone may protrude through the skin; or
- complicated: where damage may occur to internal organs, nerves or major blood vessels.

Fractures will result in:

- bleeding;
- damage to surrounding tissues;
- pain; and
- shock.

Survivors with fractures will have:

- pain at the site of the fracture;
- swelling, turning to bruising; and
- possible loss of function of the area or limb affected.

The signs of a fracture are:

- tenderness;
- deformity;
- unusual movement of the bones around fracture;
- some shock.

Treatment consists of:

- immobilising the fracture to prevent further damage and to ease pain; and

- treating the patient for shock and controlling the bleeding.

*All fractures should be handled gently and carefully.*

In a survival craft it is only possible to keep the injured survivor comfortable and free from pain by immobilising the fracture and giving morphine or pain relieving tablets.

With fractures of the limbs, put the limb in as comfortable a position as possible, providing movement does not cause pain. Force must not be applied and attempts should not be made to set the fracture, which can be set properly after rescue. When the limb is in a comfortable position, it must be kept there with the use of bandages, slings or splints.

For an arm or shoulder fracture, the arm should be put in a sling and bandaged to the chest.

For a broken leg, improvise a splint with a paddle, a salvaged piece of wood or, if necessary, secure the broken leg to the sound one, and bandage firmly but gently together at evenly spaced points down the length of the leg.

Splints must be firm, wide, and long enough to extend well above and below the fracture so that, if possible, the joints above and below the fracture are immobilised. Splints must be well padded with any available material to protect the skin and any bony joints and to allow the splint to fit snugly.

With fractures to parts of the body other than the limbs, the patient should be made as comfortable as possible. Fractures of the ribs can be supported by bandaging the arm to the body on the side of the fracture.

Fractures of the jaw should not be bandaged unless the patient is fully conscious, because if the airway is obstructed (e.g. by vomiting) the jaw may need to be open to clear it. A bandage can be used lightly to to give support if rescue may be delayed, but the jaw must not be held tightly closed. Where rescue is imminent, the casualty can support the jaw with a hand.

Survivors with suspected fractures of spine or pelvis should be immobilised and must be handled very carefully to prevent future paraplegy.

Any survivors suffering from fractures should be treated if possible by another survivor with first aid training experience. In moving such persons into survival craft great care must be taken to ensure that they remain as still as possible. Each injured survivor should be wedged between two other survivors to prevent him or her from rolling with the movement of the survival craft.

## Treating oil fuel contamination

Survivors may be affected by oil fuel on the water when abandoning ship, especially where they have to remain in the water for some time.

Contamination by oil fuel may result in:
swallowing oil fuel;
clogged skin pores;
polluted lungs; and
inflamed eyes.

Swallowing oil fuel will cause vomiting but will not poison a survivor. Additional water (or milk if available) should be given; the effect will wear off in a couple of days.

Oil clinging to the skin should be cleaned off using whatever is available in the survival craft. Skin clogged with oil is unable to perspire or breathe, and could be a cause of death if the survivor is totally smothered in oil. Oil soaked clothing should be streamed in water until clean.

Pollution of the lungs by oil fuel, or by the vapours given off from oil fuel, can be very dangerous and may lead to pneumonia. Little treatment can be given in survival craft.

Oil in the eyes will blur the vision and cause the eyes to sting. Eyes should be washed out and protected from bright sunlight for a day or so until the inflammation has gone.

## LONG-TERM CARE FOR SURVIVORS

All occupants of a survival craft are at risk and are likely to require medical treatment for some of the following conditions regardless of their physical state when they first board the craft.

## Hypothermia

Hypothermia is the condition of low body-core temperature. This results from prolonged heat loss due to immersion or insufficient clothing or covering in cold, wet and windy conditions. It is also associated with physical exhaustion, hunger and anxiety or low morale. All survivors, especially those in open craft, are likely to find themselves in these circumstances.

The combination of wet, wind and cold increases the probability of hypothermia in insufficiently protected survivors. The heat loss from wet skin is greater than from dry skin, and wind on unprotected skin increases the heat loss. Damp windy conditions with temperatures less than 6°C are most dangerous to unprotected survivors.

*All survivors should know that hypothermia is a killer.* Its onset can be rapid and if not recognised by the victim or other survivors, death is likely to follow within one hour. A victim of hypothermia often does not realise his or her condition so it is important that the signs of hypothermia are known. People have died of exposure without even complaining of the cold.

*Hypothermia is not easily recognisable. A victim is exhausted, reluctant to do anything, difficult to reason with and has slowed mental and physical reactions. Sense of touch is poor, speech may be slurred, and lips, hands and feet may swell.*

The only safe treatment for hypothermia is to shelter the victim from wet and wind. Warm the person with extra clothing or coverings and by contact with fit survivors, such as by having two people lie alongside him or her. On no account should the body or limbs be rubbed in an attempt to warm the victim. When survivors reach land, victims of hypothermia must not be placed close to external heat, such as a fire.

To lessen the possibility of hypothermia the basic need is shelter from wet, wind and cold. Protection from wet and wind is mainly provided by clothing, blankets, canopies of liferafts, covers of enclosed lifeboats and capsules and exposure covers of open lifeboats. Survival craft should also be kept as dry as possible, and in cold and wet weather survivors should attempt to keep their clothing dry.

Protection against cold is achieved through clothing or coverings and in enclosed craft, or craft with canopies or covers closed, by letting body heat raise the temperature of the craft. Liferaft floors, when inflated, provide insulation against cooling from the sea, and lifejackets can provide further insulation. Survivors keeping watch outside the closed portion of a survival craft should have the use of the most waterproof and windproof clothing available.

Remember, too, that survivors who have had the least physical exertion, who are best protected and who have high morale are the least likely to be affected by hypothermia.

*However, should a person be affected by hypothermia, the following measures will be necessary to preserve life:*

After rescue, first check if the person is breathing. Listen for heart sounds. If the survivor is not breathing, begin artificial respiration. Continue mouth to mouth or mouth to nose resuscitation until medical advice is available; in any case for at least half an hour.

The heart may be beating very slowly — one or two beats per minute — so check the pulse for a full minute instead of the usual five to ten seconds. Do not compress the chest if a heart beat is present, even if very slow. Sudden movement or a blow in severe cases can stop the heart (or cause ventricular fibrillation — which has the same result).

At the same time, so far as possible, and after breathing is restored:

- Prevent further heat loss due to evaporation or exposure.
- Place the survivor next to other people for warmth. Huddling together under covers will promote heat transfer to the victim.
- Avoid unnecessary handling of the person.
- When conscious, give a warm sweet drink.
- Do not wrap in a blanket unless the air temperature is less than the water temperature or unless the blankets have been preheated. (Unheated blankets insulate the cold body surface from the source of the external heat.)
- Do not massage the body or limbs.
- Do not feed solids or liquids to an unconscious survivor.
- Do not give alcohol.

## Immersion foot

This is due to the action of cold on a limb, usually caused by immersion in cold water. The feet become chilled and wet, resulting in poor circulation.

The affected part is swollen, numb and painful, and later the skin may become discoloured or broken.

If immersion foot occurs, keep the victim warm, and elevate the affected part. Warm the victim's body first, then the limbs and do not massage the feet. Relieve the victim's pain. If ulcers or blisters occur cover them with clean dressings.

To prevent survivors suffering from immersion foot keep the survival craft as dry as possible and survivors' feet as warm as possible.

Any shoes and socks should be removed at intervals, the feet dried and the legs and feet exercised as far as possible by making full knee and ankle movements.

If the feet begin to swell take off any footwear and wrap the feet in dry clothing material or warm them in the laps of other survivors.

## Frostbite

This is a more severe form of injury due to freezing temperatures and will only occur if the wind is allowed to play on exposed skin. The areas most likely to be affected are the face, ears and hands.

Signs of frostbite are a dirty white, waxy appearance and numbness of the skin.

The chance of survivors being affected by frostbite are slight but should survivors experience very cold conditions they should keep all areas likely to be affected covered as much as possible when they are outside canopies, covers, etc. They should watch each other's faces for the tell-tale white patches.

To treat frostbite keep the victim warm and keep the affected area warm with the hands or warm material. The affected area should be handled gently and should not be moved about or massaged in any way until thawing is complete.

## Sunburn

People doing duty in the open, such as lookouts, should take care to cover up as much of their skin as possible to prevent sunburn, and use 15 plus sunscreen. Other survivors should keep out of the sun as far as possible.

Because of the conditions in survival craft, survivors are more susceptible to sunburn. This is likely to lead to blistering and risk of infection.

Sunburn should be treated as a mild burn. Do not prick any blisters but apply a sunscreen, if available – if blisters are broken there is some risk of infection. The burn should be managed as for any other burn. Sunscreens serve the same purpose as the paraffin gauze dressings and also make a good substitute.

## Salt water boils and sores

These are likely to occur when survivors' skins are saturated with salt water, such as when sitting in water in survival craft. Skin sodden with salt water is not resistant to infection in small cuts and scratches.

Do not squeeze boils or sores but cover with antiseptic cream and dressings and leave to heal. However if the skin is kept wet, it will break down. Use Betadine (if available) rather than cream to help keep it dry.

Chafing sores are likely to form on buttocks after several days in survival craft.

## Body functions

### Urine

All survivors should urinate within the first couple of hours in a survival craft, and at least once more during the first day, as shock and hypothermia can cause muscles to seize. This could have serious consequences as the kidneys will continue producing urine, and appropriate medical treatment is not possible in a lifeboat or liferaft.

There is no benefit from retaining urine in the bladder as water cannot be resorbed from urine in this organ into the general circulation.

With no water ration given on the first day except to the sick or injured, and the small ration on following days, the amount of urine will decrease especially after the third or fourth day, and it will become harder to pass. The urine will also become darker in colour and thicker as the amount of water in the body decreases.

Urination will be increased and will be made easier if the water supply is supplemented by rainwater, dew, condensation, etc.

### Bowel movements

Survivors should not worry if they become constipated after the first couple of days. There is very little waste residue in the emergency rations in survival craft and therefore less to be passed.

In addition, constipation will prevent the loss of valuable water from the body that occurs with bowel movements.

## Dehydration

The adult human body contains about 40 litres of water, of which about 25 litres must be maintained for life to continue.

The normal amount of water lost by a resting adult each day when neither food nor water is taken is about one litre. It is proportionately more for children/babies due to the larger surface-to-volume ratio. It is important to keep covered up to reduce the loss of water from the body. A person should therefore survive for about two weeks if there is no additional loss of water.

With a minimum water ration of half a litre per day for the second, third and fourth days, a survivor should, in theory, live for at least 18 days.

However, accelerated water loss will be caused by exertion, sweating, vomiting, diarrhoea, drinking urine, drinking sea water, or eating or sucking fish. Exertion should be avoided as far as possible.

Sweating must be reduced by avoiding unnecessary activity, keeping sun off body, keeping floor of inflatable liferaft deflated, dousing canopies, covers, etc with sea water to cool interior of craft, soaking clothes during daytime for cooling from evaporation, and providing maximum through-ventilation in craft.

*Survivors should know that all the acceptable loss of water from the body could occur within 24 hours through sweating, particularly in the tropics.*

Vomiting must be avoided by taking seasickness tablets. Survivors who are seasick for more than the first day should be given additional water in small sips.

Survivors must avoid any foodstuffs likely to cause diarrhoea because of the loss of body water involved. If affected avoid food until recovered.

Urine contains poisonous waste materials dissolved in water. These waste products are of no use to the body, and urine must not be drunk.

Drinking sea water will greatly reduce the chances of survival. The salt put into the body requires more water to dissolve it for the kidneys to pass it out. This water can only be taken from the body cells, thereby increasing dehydration and increasing thirst. A vicious circle is set up, and the more sea water drunk, the greater the thirst. Continued drinking of sea water is fatal.

Survivors should avoid the temptation to use sea water for dry and cracked lips.

People attempting to drink sea water must be physically restrained for their own good. War-time experience indicates that the death rate in survival craft where salt water was drunk was seven to eight times higher than in craft where no sea water was drunk.

Eating or sucking fish, seabirds and seaweeds increases the intake of salt, to a greater or lesser degree. Seaweed and fish should never be eaten, except when the water ration has been supplemented and at least an additional litre of water is available to each survivor. The juice squeezed out of fish and birds is also rather salty, and should be supplemented by fresh water. The spinal fluid of fish, however, contains fresh water and may be safely sucked out and swallowed.

If fish are caught or seaweed collected the fleshy parts should be cut open and dried so that a store of food is built up for when rainwater can be collected.

## Delirium and mental disturbance

Delirium is most likely to be caused by drinking sea water. A delirious person will have delusions and may attempt to jump into the water. It is impossible to reason with a delirious person; restraint may be required.

Survivors suffering from exhaustion, injuries, etc, may become irrational or light-headed. They should be humoured as much as possible, but carefully watched for sudden irrational actions.

## Hygiene

Survivors should be urged to keep their skins and mouths clean.

The skin is likely to become infected from ingrained salt and dirt, and salt-covered clothing rubbing against it. Providing the temperature allows, exposure to rain water, bathing and brief exposure to sun and fresh air are likely to to be beneficial. If bathing, survivors should be attached to survival craft by lifelines and should not waste energy by swimming about. A lookout should be kept for predatory fish.

Survivors are likely to find that their lips and tongues will become swollen and their lips may crack due to the small ration of water and the lack of saliva in the mouth. The inside of the mouth is likely to become furry and foul-tasting.

Every attempt should be made to clean the inside of the mouth with a piece of cloth if necessary wrung out as dry as possible after dipping in the sea some benefit might also be obtained from sucking a button.

# Chapter 5
# Detection

## CONTENTS OF THIS CHAPTER

## ATTRACTING ATTENTION — EQUIPMENT AVAILABLE FOR ATTRACTING ATTENTION

### Emergency Position Indicating Radio Beacons (EPIRBs)

A 406 MHz satellite EPIRB transmits a distress signal to a COSPAS-SARSAT polar orbiting satellite, which relays it via a Local User Terminal (LUT) to a Maritime Rescue Coordination Centre (MRCC). The position of a 406 MHz EPIRB can be determined anywhere in the world to an accuracy of two to three miles. Depending on the relative locations of the EPIRB, the satellite, and the LUT, the time taken between switching on the EPIRB to the alert being received at an MRCC could be from a few minutes to several hours. All Australian approved 406 MHz EPIRBs also contain a 121.5 MHz transmitter for aircraft homing.

A 1.6 GHz EPIRB or 'L' band transmits a signal to an INMARSAT satellite which relays it to a coast or land earth station. The message is then relayed to an MRCC. Only polar areas (approx. outside 70° N or S) are not covered by INMARSAT satellites. The signal from a 1.6 GHz EPIRB contains information on its position. Under normal circumstances the position information is continually updated by either the ship's satnav receiver, or through its own inbuilt satnav receiver.

A 121.5/243 MHz terrestrial EPIRB also transmits a signal to the COSPAS-SARSAT satellite, but the signal can only be relayed to a LUT when the LUT and the EPIRB are both in view of the satellite. Australian and New Zealand waters are covered by the respective LUTs, as are almost all waters north of 30° N, but coverage elsewhere is patchy. The signal from a 121.5/243 MHz beacon is also receivable by any civil or military aircraft which is within range and is listening on that frequency. Searching aircraft use the signal from this EPIRB for locating survival craft.

### Portable radio equipment

This equipment is being phased out as ships are converted to GMDSS, and will not be required on any ship after 1 February 1995. This equipment can transmit on three frequencies: 500, 2182 or 8368.5 kHz. 500 and 8368.5 are Morse frequencies; 2182 is a voice frequency. Some old sets may still operate on 8364 kHz, not having been converted to 8368.5 — THEY SHOULD NOT BE USED FOR INITIAL COMMUNICATIONS ON 8364 AS THIS CHANNEL IS NO LONGER MONITORED BY COAST STATIONS.

Survivors will probably prefer to use 2182 kHz for spoken messages. However, a greater range of transmission will be achieved by the use of Morse Code on 500 or 8368.5 kHz. The Morse Code and phonetic alphabet are reproduced below.

*Morse Code*

| | | | | | |
|---|---|---|---|---|---|
| A | · — | N | — · | 1 | · — — — — |
| B | — · · · | O | — — — | 2 | · · — — — |
| C | — · — · | P | · — — · | 3 | · · · — — |
| D | — · · | Q | — — · — | 4 | · · · · — |
| E | · | R | · — · | 5 | · · · · · |
| F | · · — · | S | · · · | 6 | — · · · · |
| G | — — · | T | — | 7 | — — · · · |
| H | · · · · | U | · · — | 8 | — — — · · |
| I | · · | V | · · · — | 9 | — — — — · |
| J | · — — — | W | · — — | 0 | — — — — — |
| K | — · — | X | — · · — | | |
| L | · — · · | Y | — · — — | | |
| M | — — | Z | — — · · | | |

*Phonetic Numbers*

| | | | |
|---|---|---|---|
| 0 | Nadazero | 5 | Pantafive |
| 1 | Unaone | 6 | Soxisix |
| 2 | Bissotwo | 7 | Setteseven |
| 3 | Terrathree | 8 | Oktoeight |
| 4 | Kartefour | 9 | Novenine |

*Phonetic Alphabet*

| | | |
|---|---|---|
| Alpha | Juliet | Sierra |
| Bravo | Kilo | Tango |
| Charlie | Lima | Uniform |
| Delta | Mike | Victor |
| Echo | November | Whiske |
| Foxtrot | Oscar | X-ray |
| Golf | Papa | Yankee |
| Hotel | Quebec | Zulu |
| India | Romeo | |

## Portable two-way radiotelephone apparatus

As the primary purpose of this equipment is for communication between survival craft, between ship and survival craft, and between ship and rescue boat, their output power and therefore range under normal conditions is relatively low.

In good conditions it should be possible to contact a ship which is within sight on VHF channel 16, as all ships at sea are required to keep watch on VHF DSC and, in Australian waters, channel 16. In some circumstances, using a lifejacket whistle to signal SOS in Morse into the microphone may be heard better than the voice transmission of 'MAYDAY', but both should be tried.

## Parachute distress rockets

Parachute distress rockets, and indeed all pyrotechnics, should not be fired except on the instruction of the person in charge of the survival craft, or group of craft.

The major use of the rocket is to attract the attention of ships or aircraft at night, when the likely range of visibility is approximately 20 miles. The time taken for the red flare to drift down on its parachute allows ships or aircraft time to obtain a bearing or heading.

*During daytime the visibility from the air will be considerably reduced and aircraft flying above the flare might not even see it.* The range of visibility in daytime from ships, both of the flare and of its trailing column of smoke, should be better than from aircraft, but still lower than the night-time range.

Instructions for firing the parachute distress rocket are printed on each rocket. The rockets can be safely fired from the hand with negligible recoil. The first opportunity should be taken to read the firing instructions in order to be ready at an instant's notice.

Use parachute distress rockets to attract the attention of ships or aircraft at a distance from you. If they alter course towards you, fire another rocket to confirm the heading, and then use red hand flares as the craft comes closer. However, survivors should remember that searching aircraft may fly various patterns in search operations. It is recommended that pyrotechnics be used only when the best chance exists of their being seen by the search craft. This is usually when the search craft is heading towards the survival craft.

## Red hand flares

These signals are ideal for day or night-time use when ships or aircraft are in view. As a flare will burn for one minute it should be activated when an aircraft is estimated to be 10 miles away and heading in the general direction of the survival craft. The red flare is visible for up to five miles by day and ten or more by night in good conditions.

It is recommended that the red hand flare be used to guide approaching ships or aircraft to the survival craft, after use of EPIRBs, radio equipment, and parachute distress rockets.

When firing this signal hold it well out on the lee side of the survival craft to avoid damage by sparks which might fall from the flare. A wet cloth wrapped around the user's hand provides protection from sparks which might cause the user to drop the flare.

## Buoyant and hand-held orange smoke signals

These signals are for daytime use only. The buoyant signal produces a large amount of orange smoke for at least three minutes while the hand-held signal produces smoke for one minute only. In a light wind the smoke will make a good signal, but in moderate or strong winds the smoke is soon broken up and dispersed. Orange smoke is more easily seen from aircraft than from boats, but even in good conditions it may not be visible beyond two or three miles. The signals are particularly useful for pinpointing your location to searchers, but are of doubtful use in raising an alarm.

Instructions for activating the smoke signal are printed on the canister.

## Signalling torch

The signalling torch can be used at night together with pyrotechnics when ships or aircraft are seen, but should be used to send a simple message such as SOS. An advantage of the torch is it is directional, and so can be pointed at ships or aircraft. A flashing light is more likely to be sighted than a steady light. A battery-operated Aldis lamp is ideal for attracting attention, but care must be taken not to leak battery acid onto liferaft fabric. Unless the battery is sealed, it should be used in a lifeboat rather than a liferaft.

## Heliograph

The reflection of the sun from the heliograph mirror can be seen at a range of 20 miles in good conditions and at a lesser range under hazy conditions. On bright days it is the most effective visual signal. Instructions on its use are on the pack. Correct use according to the instructions is most important.

Its use is easiest when the sun is in front of or above the user as the target is sighted. When the sun is behind the user it is difficult, if not impossible, to use the heliograph. The speed and angle of approach of target also affect its ease of use.

Attempt to flash the reflected light onto and away from the target. Under most survival conditions the movements of craft and operator will provide sufficient flashing effect.

To attract the attention of aircraft direct flashes at high-flying aircraft, or ahead of the direction of the sound of aircraft that cannot be seen. If a search is thought to be in progress have someone flash the heliograph around the horizon at regular intervals. Use the heliograph to direct approaching aircraft to the location of survival craft.

## Radar transponders and radar reflectors

These provide pinpoint location to searching vessels, and are especially useful in conditions of poor visibility when pyrotechnics, torches and heliographs are less effective. The radar transponder is required to have a minimum range of five miles when mounted correctly in a liferaft and interrogated by a ship's radar at a scanner height of 15 metres. The range is increased when the radar scanner, and/or the transponder is at a greater height. Where possible, the transponder should be operated from a lifeboat and as high as possible, secured to an oar or boathook to get the best possible height and range. They are designed to operate in the 3 cm (9 GHz) marine radar band, and may be located by suitably equipped aircraft at ranges of up to 30 miles.

Radar reflectors, when mounted correctly in a liferaft or lifeboat, have a maximum range of about four miles.

## Other means of attracting attention

*Oil lamp.* This can be used as a steady light, or as an intermittent light when alternately shown and shielded by a bucket.

*Smoke and flames.* These can be generated by burning oil soaked rags in a bucket floated a short distance away from the survival craft, on the end of a buoyant line.

*Lights on survival craft.* The lights attached to some craft have a range of visibility of approximately two miles.

*Retro-reflective tape.* This will reflect the light shown by searchlights from searching ships or aircraft.

*Colour of canopy or exposure cover.* Under fine conditions canopies or covers of survival craft may be sighted at distances up to five miles.

*Whistles.* In certain stages of a search the use of a whistle, as provided in the survival equipment, may aid in attracting attention.

*Oil.* If it is known that an air search is under way creation of an oil slick may assist detection. Under some conditions an oil slick may be more readily visible from the air than the survival craft itself.

## ASSESSING THE SITUATION AND TAKING ACTION

Survival craft carry only a limited supply of equipment to attract attention. It is vital that this equipment is not wasted by improper use.

**If a 406 MHz or 1.6 GHz EPIRB is available** it should be activated immediately and set floating at the end of its tether line. Signals will be radiated for about two days from a 406 MHz EPIRB. From a 1.6 GHz EPIRB signals are radiated for four hours at 44-hour intervals.

After this period, one of the 121.5/243 MHz EPIRBs from the liferafts, if available, should be activated to guide search aircraft to the survival craft location.

*Nothing is to be gained by operating several EPIRBs at once; this only wastes a valuable resource.*

**If a 406 MHz or 1.6 GHz EPIRB** is not

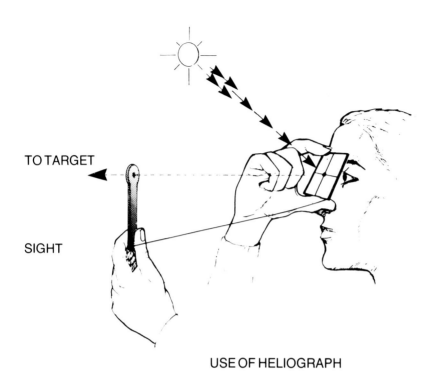

TO TARGET

SIGHT

USE OF HELIOGRAPH

APPEARANCE WHEN CORRECTLY TRAINED

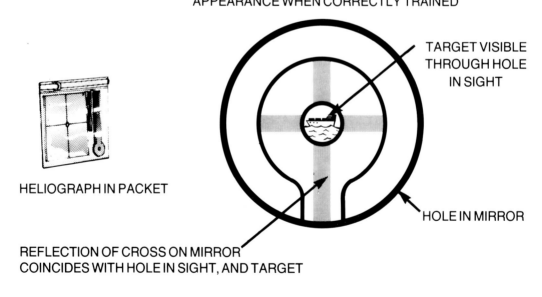

TARGET VISIBLE
THROUGH HOLE
IN SIGHT

HELIOGRAPH IN PACKET

HOLE IN MIRROR

REFLECTION OF CROSS ON MIRROR
COINCIDES WITH HOLE IN SIGHT, AND TARGET

THE HELIOGRAPH AND ITS USE

available survivors should activate one of the liferaft 121.5/243 MHz EPIRBs immediately. The system coverage area as at November 1992 is shown in the diagram on page 64.

## Radar transponders

If the ship sinks or is abandoned in a shipping lane, one radar transponder should be operated as soon as it can be secured in place in the survival craft. The battery has sufficient capacity for at least four days operation in the standby condition (when not being interrogated), and has transmission capacity for a further eight hours. Away from a shipping lane, unless it is known that a ship is in the vicinity, operation of the radar transponder should normally be delayed until it is known that searching craft are in the vicinity.

## EPIRB detection time

The detection time for a 1.6 GHz EPIRB should be approx. two minutes or less, as these should always be in sight of an INMARSAT geostationary satellite.

The *average* detection time for a 406 MHz EPIRB anywhere in the world, or a satellite compatible 121.5/243 MHz EPIRB within the 'real time' coverage area of a COSPAS-SARSAT Local User Terminal (LUT) is of the order of 90 minutes. Detection time is a function, for a 121.5/243 MHz EPIRB, of the survivors' position relative to the nearest LUT, and the current configuration of satellites relative to LUT and the EPIRB. Coverage areas for the Australian and New Zealand LUTs are shown in the diagram on p. 64. At the edge of the coverage area average detection time rapidly increases until the probability of detection by satellite becomes zero. Detection by aircraft remains possible.

## THE SEARCH PROBLEM

## Search organisation

Before a search can be mounted, the Search and Rescue (SAR) authority must first become aware that an emergency or potential emergency exists. In the event of a distress message being received a search is mounted. To this end it is essential to indicate the position of the distress so that the search area can be pin-pointed.

Three possible situations may exist with respect to the location of a SAR incident when it is reported to the SAR authorities.

### Position known (approximately)

The incident may have been witnessed, reported as a fix by a shorebased radar, direction finding network, another vessel, or by the distressed ship itself, or computed by the SAR Authority from a previously reported and reliable position of the distressed ship (this indicates the importance of reporting systems such as AUSREP and AMVER).

### Track known (approximately)

The distressed ship may have filed a sailing plan prior to its departure, which included its intended track or route, but its actual position along the intended track is unknown.

### Area known (generally)

When neither the position nor the intended track is known it may be possible (though difficult) to determine the probable area within which the survival craft may be.

Ideally, the search area will be based on the position given in a distress message, plus allowance for wind and current over the intervening period.

*Seafarers should take note of the need to participate in ship-reporting schemes, leave advice of intended track for a voyage, send distress calls and messages, together with preceding urgency call and messages if circumstances permit. The importance of alerting a coast radio station at the first sign of trouble cannot be over-estimated. After abandoning ship, survivors must reduce drift to a minimum to reduce the probable search area.*

## Search methods

### Visual

This is the oldest as well as the most commonly used method for detecting distressed craft or persons. As a result it has benefited from an extensive amount of research and practical testing. The detectability of a target is relative to size, shape, distance, brightness and colour contrast with the background, its movement and the length of time seen by an observer.

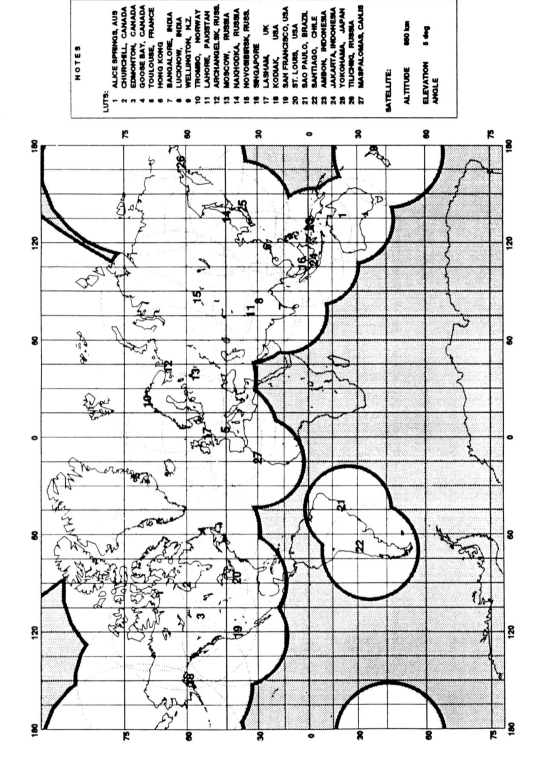

SATELLITE VISIBILITY FOR SATELLITE COMPATIBLE    121.5/243 MHz EPIRBs

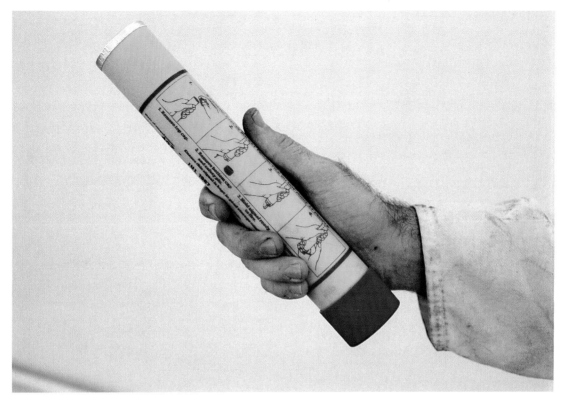

HAND-HELD FLARE SHOWING FIRING INSTRUCTIONS

## Electronic

*Electronic*

This includes using radar and radio. Under proper conditions electronic searches are far more efficient than visual searches. Relatively large track spacings can be used and, as a result, a higher probability of detection can be obtained over a larger geographical area in a shorter period of time.

## The search

According to the data available a search will be carried out by ships or aircraft or both.

When a distress message is transmitted giving a position, ships in or approaching the area will divert to give assistance. The early use of aircraft will depend on the distance of survivors from the coast and from airfields.

When a ship is known to have EPIRBs aboard an early electronic search by air may be planned to detect signals from the beacon. If no distress messages or other transmissions are heard visual searches may involve many ships and aircraft.

Aircraft carrying out an electronic search for signals from an EPIRB will most likely be flying at a medium height of 10,000 ft. Aircraft conducting visual searches will fly low, at 500 to 1000 ft.

If signals from an EPIRB are heard by a search aircraft it will attempt to establish your position by flying at a constant range around you. It will then close in, or direct another aircraft in, to make a visual sighting. Do not worry if the aircraft then flies off — it is probably going to direct a search ship towards your position. Do not switch your EPIRB off at this stage — it may be needed to relocate you.

Aircraft searching visually at night will fire a green flare approximately every five minutes, and at each turning point on their search pattern. On sighting a green flare you should:

- wait until the green flare has died, then fire a rocket or hand flare;
- wait a further one minute, then fire a second rocket or flare. The aircraft will acknowledge

sighting these flares by firing a succession of green flares and switching on its landing lights;

- if it is believed the aircraft is not heading directly towards you fire further single rockets or flares to guide the aircraft;
- when the aircraft is about one mile away, fire a further rocket or flare and then protect your eyes from the glare of the aircraft searchlight which may be used to identify the contact.

Should there not be enough flares to carry out all the above procedures the following points should be observed carefully:

- The first rocket or flare should not be fired until the aircraft's flare has completely died.
- A second rocket or flare should not be fired until a full minute after the first flare.
- If only one rocket or flare then remains this should be saved until the aircraft is within two miles or until just before it passes abeam.

After locating survivors aircraft may drop survival equipment. This can vary from a 'helibox' (a cardboard box which rotates on folding fins as it falls) or a 'storepedo' (a styrofoam container with communications equipment, equipment to mark the position of food/water, etc.) to sea rescue kits. These latter consist of up to five cylindrical containers linked together with buoyant rope coloured bright orange.

The kits can comprise a single container (a liferaft) or a string, normally with liferafts at each end and containers of supplies and equipment in between. The liferafts are usually 10-person size, and will commence inflating as they leave the aircraft. When deployed on the water the overall length of the string may be up to 550 metres. For multiple container drops including liferafts, pilots will drop the equipment slightly upwind of survivors in the water or on buoyant apparatus, and slightly downwind of survivors in inflatable liferafts, allowing the equipment to drift to survivors and vice versa.

Military aircraft may also drop SAR Datum Buoys or Sonobuoys to mark the position of the survivors for aircraft homing. On impact Sonobuoys release a small hydrophone which hangs under the Sonobuoy on a light cable. If no other means of communication is available the hydrophone may be retrieved and used as a microphone for one-way communication to the aircraft. The Sonobuoy must be left floating in the water.

# Chapter 6
# Retrieval

This chapter is concerned with the safe and speedy rescue of survivors.

Rescuing of survivors from their survival craft will most likely be made by a ship or a smaller vessel. However, in certain cases the recovery of survivors by helicopter is possible.

## CONTENTS OF THIS CHAPTER

## RESCUE BY SHIP

While the major part of a search for survivors may be conducted from the air, most survivors are rescued by ships. Both naval and merchant ships may be involved in a search, in which case the ship best fitted to achieve a recovery will be detailed. In other cases survivors may be rescued by passing ships not involved in the search.

Removing survivors from their survival craft to the safety of the rescue ship is a very difficult phase of the whole life-saving incident. It is likely that the survivors are unable to help themselves to safety. In the majority of cases survivors will have to be assisted or even hoisted on board the ship.

Depending on the weather, light, depth of water, sea condition and the rescue ship's size and ability to manoeuvre, the ship may stop close to the survival craft and launch a lifeboat or a rescue boat to recover survivors, float down a liferaft on a line, or fire, throw or trail a line down to survival craft.

The smaller the ship and the lower its freeboard, the easier it is to come alongside survival craft to assist people directly aboard.

The ship or small boat may tow survival craft into more sheltered water before recovering survivors. Survivors should note that rescue ships may release vegetable or animal oils to reduce the effect of the waves before carrying out the rescue.

As sea anchors from survival craft may foul sea suctions, transducers, fins, bilge keels or propellers of the rescuing ship, survivors should be ready to retrieve sea anchors before the rescue ship comes alongside.

## RESCUE BY HELICOPTER

Although helicopters vary in speed, range of operations and the number of people who can be carried, the operation is similar.

Shore-based helicopters can operate up to a maximum of 150 miles from the coast, but at that distance, because of limited fuel capacity, they would not be able to remain on station very long before returning to base. They are subject to certain operational limitations. Unless they are dedicated Search and Rescue Helicopters, they normally cannot effect a pickup at sea by night, and may be unable to recover survivors in heavy seas.

Naval helicopters are well practised in rescuing survivors from a small craft or the sea by day and night. The methods noted below are used:

- *Rescue net.* The rescue net has a conically shaped 'bird cage' appearance and is open on one side (see diagram on page 68). When the net is trailing in the water its opening is stabilised by the use of a drogue. The survivor enters the opening, sits in the net and holds on.

- *Litter (stretcher).* Injured persons should be evacuated in the litter provided by the helicopter. This is rigged with the proper bridles and means for attaching to the hoist cable.

- *Rescue sling (strop).* This device, although efficient, is the most troublesome for persons not familiar with its use. Survivors should therefore note the proper procedure. Used properly it is quick and nearly foolproof.

*Rescue from a survival craft.* If an assistant is available, he or she should hold the sling like a coat being held for someone to don. The survivor to be hoisted merely backs up to it, inserts one arm, followed by head and trunk and then the other arm, drops his arms to his waist, and clasps one wrist with the other hand.

The two paramount rules are:

- Do not sit in the sling.

- Keep the yoke of the sling and the hoist cable to the front.

When used in this manner the survivor will not fall from the sling while being hoisted, even if he or she loses consciousness.

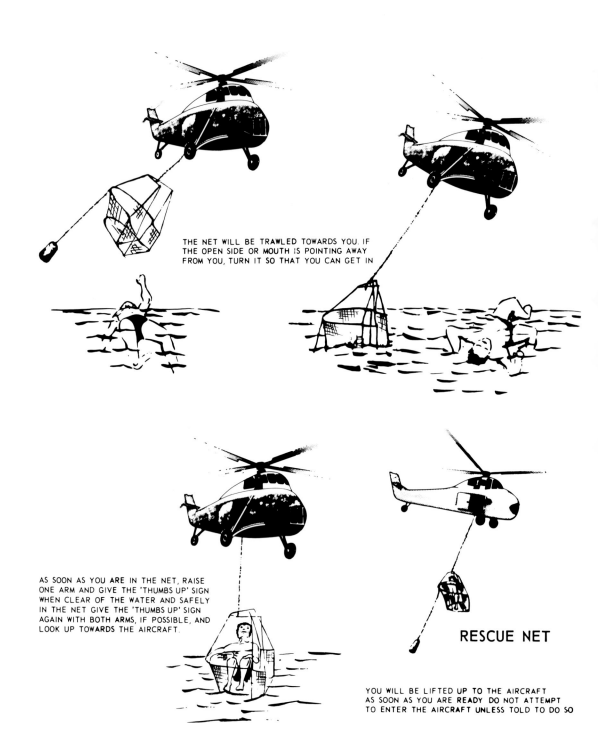

THE NET WILL BE TRAWLED TOWARDS YOU. IF
THE OPEN SIDE OR MOUTH IS POINTING AWAY
FROM YOU, TURN IT SO THAT YOU CAN GET IN

AS SOON AS YOU ARE IN THE NET, RAISE
ONE ARM AND GIVE THE 'THUMBS UP' SIGN
WHEN CLEAR OF THE WATER AND SAFELY
IN THE NET GIVE THE 'THUMBS UP' SIGN
AGAIN WITH BOTH ARMS, IF POSSIBLE, AND
LOOK UP TOWARDS THE AIRCRAFT.

RESCUE NET

YOU WILL BE LIFTED UP TO THE AIRCRAFT
AS SOON AS YOU ARE READY DO NOT ATTEMPT
TO ENTER THE AIRCRAFT UNLESS TOLD TO DO SO

HELICOPTER RESCUE USING RESCUE NET

When there is no one to assist, the survivor should enter the sling as if it were a coat. One arm is inserted, followed by the head and trunk, and then the second arm. A slight twisting motion is required — just as one would twist when putting a coat on alone.

Should weather conditions permit, rescue by helicopter from an inflatable liferaft may be expedited by sitting on top of the canopy with or without the arch deflated.

*Rescue from the water.* The sling should be entered as follows:

* Approach the sling from the bottom or loop end (opposite the cable attachment).

* Insert one arm up from under the sling.

* Lower the head and other arm under the water and bring them up inside the loop. The sides of the sling are then under the armpits and the loop is across the back.

* Bring the hands together under the water and clasp one wrist.

It may prove difficult to don the sling in this way while a survivor is wearing a lifejacket. In this case it is preferable to grasp the hoisting cable with one hand and hold the strap with the other. Then put the feet through the strap and slip it up the body until it jams against the lifejacket behind the chest, or against the armpits.

DANGER: While in the water, hydrostatic pressure on the legs, especially if floating vertically, improves the blood supply to the head. On being lifted out, the reduction in pressure causes a drop in blood supply to the brain. BEFORE BEING RAISED THE SURVIVOR SHOULD ASSUME A HORIZONTAL POSITION TO REDUCE THE DELETERIOUS EFFECTS OF HYDROSTATIC PRESSURE REDUCTION WHEN BEING LIFTED FROM THE WATER.

Hand signals are fastest and most easily understood.

DO NOT HOIST, NOT READY: Arms extended horizontally, fingers clenched, thumbs down.
HOIST: Arms raised above the horizontal, thumbs up.

When using the rescue net or sling, the last person should hold on or position his or her arms as previously instructed and vigorously nod the head up and down when ready for hoisting.

Do not attempt to get out of the device before you are inside the helicopter. The helicopter crew member will stop the hoist, turn you as required (to face away from the door) and pull you down and into the cabin. The person being hoisted should not attempt to assist in any way unless so instructed. The crew member is well trained. If more than one person is to be hoisted, the first, who may be required to assist the hoist operator in embarking others, must do no more than instructed.

Helicopters used for search and rescue are fitted with UHF and VHF communications equipment, M/F radio compass and normally UHF homing equipment.

If survivors see that the helicopter is going to pass by, or is on a course which will take it away, continued use should be made of visual distress signals while at the same time, using the portable radio, reporting the fact to the coast station, stating the present bearing and distance of the helicopter. The coast station will pass this information to the helicopter.

## RESCUE BY BREECHES BUOY

In some countries life-saving organisations use the Breeches Buoy and Rocket Life Saving Apparatus to rescue people.

A rocket with a line attached is fired across the ship. Secure the line to a firm point on the ship. Having done so, signal to the shore personnel. The latter will then bend an endless fall and a tail block to the rocket line. When you receive an affirmative signal from the shore, haul on the rocket line until you receive the tail block and endless fall.

Make the tail block fast to a convenient position, clear of obstructions, and remove the rocket line. Give an affirmative signal to the shore. The shore personnel will then bend a hawser to one part of the endless fall (the whip), and haul it off to the ship.

Make fast this hawser to the same part of the ship as the tail block is made fast to, but above it. Make sure that the hawser is clear of the whip. Then give the affirmative signal to the shore.

The shore personnel will then set the hawser taut, and send a Breeches Buoy to the ship using the whip. The Buoy should be used to send persons off the ship. Each survivor should sit well down in the Breeches Buoy, and when secure the person in charge should signal the shore. The personnel on shore will haul each person ashore in this manner. The procedure is repeated until all persons are landed.

It may sometimes happen that the state of the weather and the condition of the ship may not permit a hawser to be set up. In such circumstances the Breeches Buoy will be hauled off by the whip alone.

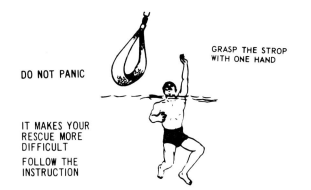

DO NOT PANIC

IT MAKES YOUR
RESCUE MORE
DIFFICULT

FOLLOW THE
INSTRUCTION

GRASP THE STROP
WITH ONE HAND

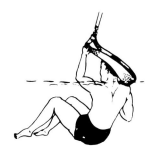

ALWAYS RETAIN A HOLD ON THE STROP
WITH ONE HAND UNTIL IT IS FITTED

SLIP THE OTHER ARM AND
THE HEAD THROUGH THE LOOP

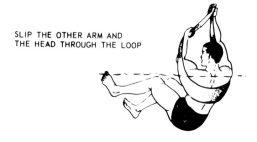

ARRANGE THE STROP SO THAT IT
FITS UNDER THE ARMPITS

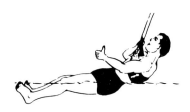

PULL THE WEBBING LOOP DOWN SO THAT IT IS AS
CLOSE AS POSSIBLE TO THE CHEST. GRASP THE
STROP WITH ONE HAND AND EXTEND THE ARM
HORIZONTALLY GIVING THE 'THUMBS UP' SIGN.
LOOK UP TOWARDS THE AIRCRAFT.

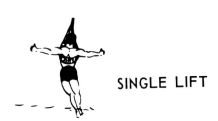

SINGLE LIFT

WHEN CLEAR OF THE WATER EXTEND BOTH ARMS HORIZONTALLY
AND GIVE THE 'THUMBS UP' SIGN. IF YOU COMMENCE TO SWING
DURING WINCHING, HOISTING MAY CEASE UNTIL THE SWING IS
BROUGHT UNDER CONTROL. WHEN AT THE HELICOPTER DOOR DO
NOT ATTEMPT TO CLIMB IN. THE CREWMAN WILL TURN YOU TO
FACE AWAY FROM THE HELICOPTER AND WILL THEN LOWER YOU
DOWN THROUGH THE DOORWAY.

## HELICOPTER RESCUE USING RESCUE SLING — SINGLE LIFT

70

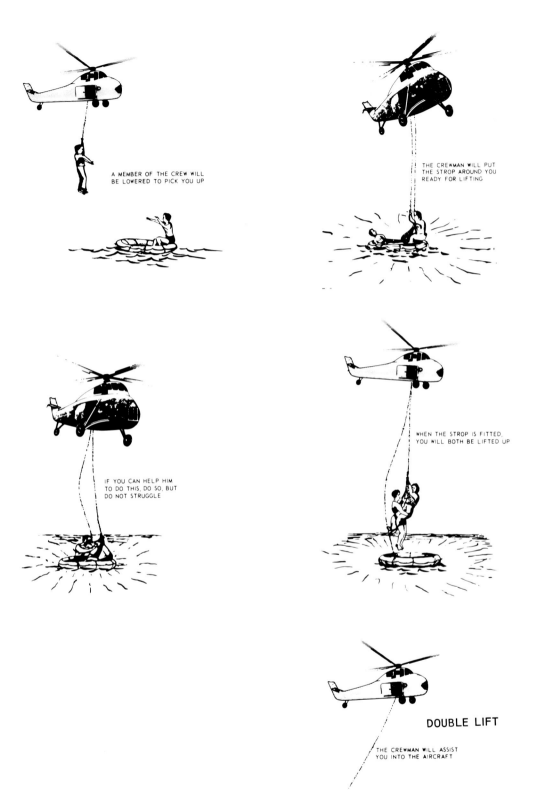

A MEMBER OF THE CREW WILL
BE LOWERED TO PICK YOU UP

THE CREWMAN WILL PUT
THE STROP AROUND YOU
READY FOR LIFTING

IF YOU CAN HELP HIM
TO DO THIS, DO SO, BUT
DO NOT STRUGGLE

WHEN THE STROP IS FITTED,
YOU WILL BOTH BE LIFTED UP

DOUBLE LIFT

THE CREWMAN WILL ASSIST
YOU INTO THE AIRCRAFT

HELICOPTER RESCUE USING RESCUE SLING — DOUBLE LIFT

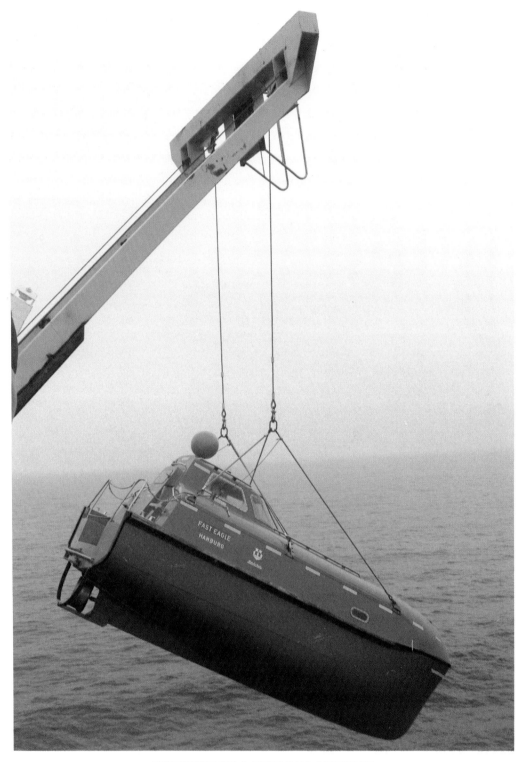

RECOVERY OF A FREE-FALL LIFEBOAT
Courtesy: Robert Hatecke Stader Bootswerft

## AFTER RESCUE

Once survivors are aboard a rescue ship or are landed from a rescue helicopter it is important to check that everyone has been rescued. While survivors will be given all available care and attention, it is necessary that a limited debriefing be conducted at an early stage to determine:

- the total complement of the abandoned ship;
- the possibility of other survivors being unaccounted for, and any information which may lead to their rescue; and
- the extent of any medical care while in survival craft, and any drugs taken.

Later, survivors will be questioned about their experiences during the survival, search, and rescue phases of the life-saving incident. Information will also be sought about the cause of the casualty to the ship. To assist the authorities all survivors can expect to be asked to complete a debriefing form (in the form of a questionnaire) in due course. The value of any notes or log kept during the time in survival craft should be self-evident.

*Note*: The Seafarers' Assistance Service is available in every State for confidential counselling for survivors. Contact 02 264 7488 for details of the nearest office.

## RECOVERY OF SURVIVAL CRAFT AND RESCUE BOATS

### Recovering a lifeboat

- Rig a boat rope along the ship's side.
- Slack down falls to the correct height for hooking on.
- Rig fenders overside.
- Make a lee for boat to come alongside the ship.
- Spread wave oil to reduce wave-breaking (if necessary).
- Boat approaches vessel; uses boat rope to keep boat alongside.
- Position boat below falls. Make fast painter.

Turn blocks to remove twists in falls.

Hook on forward fall first, and then after fall (forward here refers to direction of motion of ship through water; persons should not stand forward of forward block or abaft after block). (Persons operating outside the boat should always wear safety belts attached to strong points.)

Hold on to lifelines. (Lifelines are not always fitted where davits hold totally enclosed boats,

crew should hold fast to the boat in case of accidents and MUST WEAR THEIR SAFETY BELTS.)

- Leave operating crew in boat. In rough weather it may be preferable for the remaining people to come aboard by lifeboat ladder but only if they can do so safely, to reduce the strain on the gear and the severity of any accident but in calm weather it is preferable for full crew to come up with the boat.
- Hoist boat out of water. When well clear of water, remove plug to drain bilge water.
- When the boat is hoisted to the boat deck level, stop hoisting and fit tricing pendants.
- Lower boat slightly to allow boat to come close alongside.
- Disembark operating crew.
- Hoist boat to full height.
- When the boat has reached the stowage position, cut-off switches will cut off power to prevent the davits coming against the stops, thus preventing overstressing of the falls. If necessary hoist the boat manually to the housed position. Secure the boat by putting on gripes. Rig triggers.

*Note*: Marine Orders Part 25, Issue 1, requires passenger ships to carry rope pennants which can be attached to the lower blocks to enable an emergency boat to be hooked on and hoisted safely in a seaway, and wire pennants which can be hung from the davit heads and used to temporarily suspend the boat while the falls are overhauled. Issue 2 requires the same equipment for lifeboats used as rescue boats. The pennants should normally be of nylon, in view of its greater strength and stretching capability than other commonly used ropes.

In rough weather it may be difficult to recover and stow a survival craft in its usual stowed position. In such circumstances, a craft could perhaps be hoisted by the ship's crane or derrick. It should then be temporarily secured in a safe place on deck, till it can be housed properly. If this is not practicable consideration should be given to towing the boat till the weather allows recovery.

### Recovering a davit-launched liferaft

- Paddle to ship and pick up boat rope, or heaving line. With the aid of boat rope or line, come alongside and under the falls.
- Weather permitting, some people may climb the liferaft ladder and go on board to reduce the mass of raft while lifting.

- Lower hoisting wire to liferaft.
- Hook on liferaft.
- Hoist liferaft.
- When raft is in position just clear of the boat deck, cease hoisting. With the aid of guys, or by motor, if power-driven, slew davit and bring liferaft inboard.
- Lower liferaft on to deck.
- Disembark personnel.

*Note:* The liferaft should be sent ashore for servicing at the first opportunity.

### Recovering a rigid or an inflatable liferaft

It is unusual for a liferaft to be launched in circumstances other than abandoning ship. However should a liferaft be launched in an emergency e.g. to pick up a person floating in the water, the liferaft should be recovered. An inflated liferaft should be kept inflated, if possible, until the next port where it can be serviced in a proper manner. If it is not practical to keep the raft inflated it should be deflated and stowed away carefully until it can be landed for servicing. Since the painter of a SOLAS liferaft has a breaking tension in excess of 750 kgwt, and the mass of an empty raft, including container and equipment, is unlikely to exceed 185 kg, it should be possible to bend the remnant of the painter to a rope and lift the *empty* raft aboard a vessel. Allow water in the raft or in the water pockets to drain before heaving clear of the water.

### Recovering a free-fall lifeboat

- Position lifeboat astern of vessel.
- Slew gantry crane aft.
- Lower the fall to the water.
- Ensure crew are strapped on to seats. (Weather permitting, most of the crew can come up the ship's side by ladders rigged for the purpose, or by liferaft ladders).
- Hook on the boat.
- Hoist the boat.
- Boat will come up angled.
- Align boat with the ramp.
- Hoist gantry to bring boat onto the ramp.
- Hoist ramp to the stowed position.
- Engage locking mechanism.
- Disembark personnel.

*Note:* This will be practical in conditions approaching a flat calm only. In any other conditions it will probably be better to tow the boat into port, if possible.

### Recovering a rescue boat

This applies to approved rescue boats fitted to new ships, or retrofitted to existing ships. It does not apply to rescue boats fitted to older ships. A new ship must be able to rapidly recover a rescue boat when loaded with its full complement of people and equipment. The manufacturer's instruction book should be consulted and thoroughly understood. Recovery of the rescue boat should be practised in worsening conditions until the rescue boat crew are competent to launch the boat, pick up survivors and recover the boat in severe conditions.

# Chapter 7
# Survival on land

It is always possible that survivors may reach land before being detected, particularly if abandonment takes place in coastal waters. The problems of survival on land are similar to the problems of survival at sea, but vary according to the time which survivors have spent in survival craft and their fitness, morale, equipment and rations.

The benefits of reaching land and the needs for survival on land vary according to the location and type of land reached, its temperature and rainfall, and whether it is inhabited or not. The coastline of Australia itself represents a great variety of conditions of temperature, rainfall, habitation, etc.

As a general rule, the larger the island or land mass on which survivors land, the greater the chance of finding fresh water, food and inhabitants, and therefore of survival and eventual rescue.

## CONTENTS OF THIS CHAPTER

**Making a safe landing**
   Breakers
   Coral reefs
   Rocks
   Cliffs
   Tidal currents and rips
**Shelter**
**Water and food**
**Attracting attention**
**Exploration**
**Rescue**

The following guidelines should be varied, according to the conditions survivors find.

## MAKING A SAFE LANDING

It is essential for survivors to be able to get ashore safely without losing their craft, equipment, etc. The major hazards in getting ashore safely are breakers, coral reefs, rocks, cliffs, and tidal currents and rips. These hazards may occur together in various combinations.

## Breakers

Before attempting to land through surf, survivors should, if necessary, attempt to hold a position outside the breaker line for a short time to study the surf, height and breadth of breakers, the angle at which they strike the beach, and the effects of any rip currents (as shown by confused water, foam belts, discoloured water, gaps in the line of breakers,

and the drift of flotsam). Survivors should land as soon as is reasonable.

Before beginning to run in, survivors should pack away all loose gear or secure it to the survival craft, so that if the craft is capsized the gear will not be lost.

To beach an oar propelled lifeboat, the following procedure is recommended:

- Man the oars.
- Unship the tiller and rudder, and ship steering oar.
- Bring boat head to wind and sea, and stream sea anchor over the bow.
- Between waves, back water, with the sea anchor tripped.
- At each wave crest allow the sea anchor to grip, and row into the wave, or hold water with the blades deep.
- On shallow beach, beach stern first, and disembark over stern, taking care not to be caught by undertow.
- On steep beach, beach boat side on and disembark as quickly as possible from the ends or the seaward side of the boat. If the boat is rolled this lessens the chance of being injured or trapped by the boat.
- Pull boat as far up beach as possible.

*Note:* if possible avoid landing on a steep-to beach.

For totally enclosed boats, and motor boats generally, stream the sea anchor over the stern if possible and beach bow first under power. As far as possible the boat should be kept on the back of the wave or in the succeeding trough, with the sea anchor tripped. On the approach of the next breaking crest it is desirable to slow the engine and allow the sea anchor to 'bite', holding the stern up to the crest, while the crest passes. Full power can be used at the appropriate time to prevent the boat broaching to. The boat *must* be kept at right angles to the line of the crests.

With liferafts it is essential to keep all people as low as possible in the raft, and have both drogues streamed to hold the raft into the breakers. When beached, the raft must quickly be carried up the beach to a sheltered position.

Survivors should be aware that when a swell or waves move into a bay or cove, the seas move further inshore in the centre of the bay before breaking, so that the line of breakers becomes curved towards the shore. It may therefore be better to attempt to land on the sides of a bay to seaward of the line of breakers rather than to attempt to land at the head of the bay. Similarly, if breakers are approaching the coast at an angle, the best place to land is likely to be in the lee of any point or headland.

## Coral reefs

Coral reefs are found fringing the land masses and islands in tropical waters within the latitudes 30°N to 30°S. Common features of such reefs are a seaward slope, a reef crest extending above low tide level, a reef flat just below low tide level and a boulder zone on the inside of reef which is above low tide level. A reef may be connected directly to land or may be separated by a narrow channel of water or a wide lagoon. Many reefs form on the top of submerged mountains so that only a lagoon is seen surrounded by reefs.

Survivors should only attempt to cross reefs or find the opening to a lagoon where there is land extending well above the high water level to give sufficient protection.

Openings in reefs fringing islands are most likely due to the run-off from fresh water streams, as coral will only grow in salt water. Such passages are easily noticed when any sea is running as they will be clear of breakers.

Always try to manoeuvre survival craft towards such a safe passage. At high tide it may be possible for liferafts to be carried across the reef into the lagoon.

Because coral is sharp and can cause severe wounds, survivors should put on as much clothing as possible, including lifejackets and shoes, and should protect hands with strips of cloth.

## Rocks

Survivors should attempt to manoeuvre survival craft away from rocks extending seawards from points of land, cliffs, etc. Rocks offshore are more dangerous than those close inshore, as craft can be wrecked or capsized well away from the shore, with little chance of saving equipment.

It is likely that liferafts could be carried safely over submerged rocks by wind and waves where a lifeboat would be damaged. When approaching shore with any survival craft keep a close lookout for rocks, particularly those just submerged. Keep a paddle or boat hook hand for fending off.

## Cliffs

Survivors should keep away from high cliffs which may be difficult, if not impossible, to climb even if survivors are fit enough to do so. The base of a cliff usually provides no shelter or aids to survival.

If land is reached in the vicinity of cliffs, survivors must try to manoeuvre along the coast until the cliffs are lower or an inlet or cove is found.

Cliffs can lessen the chance of being seen by search aircraft.

## Tidal currents and rips

Although tidal streams mostly flow along a coast line, they may be pulled into bays or thrown out to seaward by major headlands. As such, they may hinder attempts to land, and may carry survivors past suitable landing places. Tidal streams will most likely be too wide for survivors to manoeuvre craft across them unless lifeboat or rescue boat motors can be used.

As tidal streams are likely to produce stronger tidal currents in narrow straits or channels, these should be avoided by survivors.

Under certain surf and beach conditions rip currents may be produced. These are distinguished by discoloured water in the rip, confused surf, gaps in breakers, flotsam carried seaward, breakers further to seaward, etc. Rip currents which start inshore with a narrow breadth of 15 to 30 metres fan out as they extend offshore for distances of up to 1000 metres. Survivors must keep a good lookout for such rips, and should do everything possible to avoid them.

The best chance of avoiding such hazards and therefore of making a safe landing will be when motor lifeboats or rescue boats are present either to land by themselves or to tow other survival craft behind them. Therefore it is important that some fuel is kept for such a need, and that the engines are maintained throughout any survival period.

## SHELTER

Survivors will need protection from the sun during the day and will need to be warm and dry at night. Protection from flies, mosquitoes, etc. is also an advantage. The ability to provide such shelter will depend upon the condition of the survival craft after reaching land and the amount of equipment retained.

If in good condition liferafts should be pulled well above high water level and lashed to trees, rocks, etc. so that they cannot be blown over. If possible lay leaves, ferns, etc. beneath raft floors for insulation. The rafts can then be used as tents.

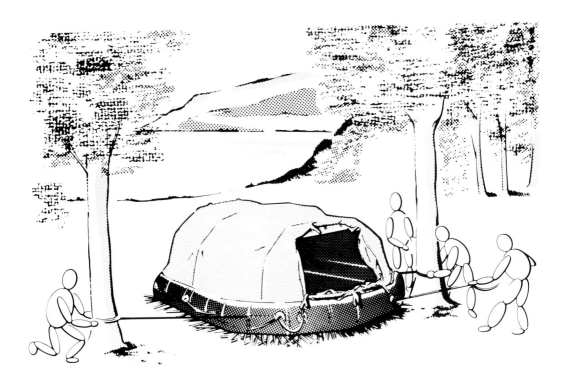

USING THE RAFT FOR SHELTER ON LAND

For survivors with lifeboats, if possible pull the boats up the beach and secure to trees or rocks. It may be preferable to remove the exposure covers of lifeboats for use as a sleeping tents, with the hoops pushed into the beach. If possible, always try to sleep at a level raised above the beach or ground.

With the use of a knife or an axe it should be possible to gather enough branches to form a simple shelter or lean-to for protection and a platform above ground level for stores and equipment.

Ideally, liferafts or other shelters should be placed on rising ground and to windward of vegetation or stagnant water to minimise the problem of mosquitoes and other insects. Avoid rotting vegetation as this may be a source of snakes and harmful insects, and do not place shelters under coconut trees because of the danger from falling nuts.

## WATER AND FOOD

For an island or area of land to be habitable, there must be a source of fresh water. If the land is, or appears to be, uninhabited, it is essential to find fresh water.

If rivers, streams or springs cannot be found it may be necessary to dig for water, using whatever means are available. Water fit to drink can often be obtained by digging a hole at least 50 to 100 metres inshore of the high water level, usually at the base of a large sandhill. The water is likely to be brackish, so dig no deeper than necessary — it will be sufficient to go 30 cm deeper after water is first found. If possible, line the hole with stones, etc. to prevent the side falling in. The fresh water will float on top of any salt water, and may be skimmed off. If the water is very brackish, try a new hole further inland.

Brackish water in small quantities is not harmful, but if a fire can be started, it is safer to boil all water collected in this way. Fresh water can be produced from salt water by an improvised still. Salt water is boiled in a bucket covered by a cloth that has been soaked in the sea and wrung out. Steam condenses in the cloth which is wrung out a number of times until all trace of salt is gone. The boiling is continued; wring out the fresh water in the cloth into a holding container.

Another possibility is the use of an improvised solar still. For this survivors can use a bucket, or dig a hole in the ground and line it with absorbent material.

## AN IMPROVISED SOLAR STILL

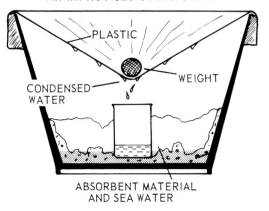

Pour a small amount of sea water into the bottom of your 'still' and in the centre of the base stand a small container to collect the condensed fresh water. Cover the 'still' with a plastic sheet, putting a weight onto the plastic directly above the collecting tin or jar.

Fresh water evaporated out of salt or brackish water will rise and condense on the plastic, running down to the lowest point and dripping into the collection bin.

A device of this type could produce a daily ration for up to 12 survivors if it is constantly tended and 'fed' with sea water.

It may also be possible to gather water from short sections of roots or the stems and leaves of plants, and coconut milk is drinkable, if coconuts are present. Avoid using any roots or stems which exude white sap or whose juice burns the mouth.

Unless a plentiful source of drinking water is found, continue attempts to collect rainwater using canopies and covers.

The sources of food available will vary considerably with the climate and conditions, but are likely to include fruits, coconuts, fish and small animals or birds.

Care must be exercised in eating fruits, particularly those that are unfamiliar. A good test for the edibility of fruit is to rub a little of the juice on the inside of the lower lip. Avoid anything that has a stinging, acid or bitter taste or anything with a milky sap. Know that birds can eat berries or fruits that are harmful to man.

As well as the flesh of the coconut being edible, the flesh can also be crushed to provide a basic form of oil for use as protection against sunburn and for use in a lamp.

The fish in coastal waters, particularly in the tropics, include poisonous and dangerous types, and care must therefore be taken when fishing and when walking or standing in the sea and in rock pools. Where fish are plentiful, they may be speared with spears cut from available timber or may be clubbed if near the surface. Any fish caught should be cooked as soon as possible.

Most shellfish are edible, but beware of those that look like cones or pointed spindles as these contain creatures with very poisonous bites. Any shellfish found should preferably be gutted and dried or cooked before eating.

Turtles may be found in some places. These may be killed for their meat and their blood. Look for trails across the beach to the places where their eggs are hidden in the sand, usually about 50cm down and about 20 metres from the water. These eggs are a good source of nourishment (see p. 42).

Look for edible vegetation in small plants and leaves. On a barren island, the only edible vegetation is likely to be pigweed, a fleshy, soft-stemmed reddish-green weed with yellow flowers, which grows in large patches. This plant will also relieve thirst.

Look for trails of small animals and improvise traps or snares to catch them. Above all, you will have to improvise using the equipment available from survival craft, and using whatever you can find ashore.

## ATTRACTING ATTENTION

Not only will the equipment from survival craft still be available for attracting attention but survivors may be able to gather sufficient fuel for a fire and materials to lay out signals or signs on the ground for sighting from the air.

A fire should be started with the matches from lifeboat or liferaft survival kits and should be kept going throughout the time ashore. This will be required for cooking food and boiling fresh water as well as for attracting attention, while it will also be a source of warmth at night.

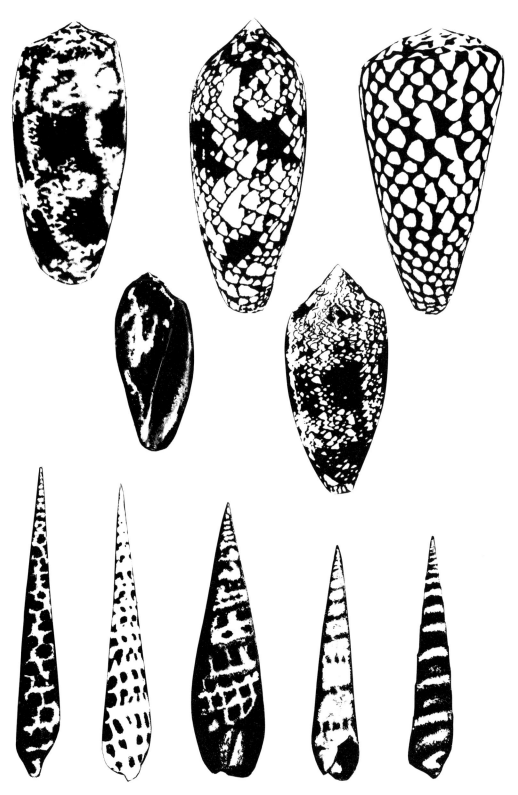

DANGEROUS SHELLFISH

## GROUND - AIR EMERGENCY CODE

| | | | | | |
|---|---|---|---|---|---|
| **I** | **II** | **X** | **F** | **≋** | **K** |
| 1. Require doctor - serious injures | 2. Require medical supplies | 3. Unable to proceed | 4. Require food and water | 5. Require firearms and ammunition | 6. Indicate direction and proceed |
| **↑** | | | | **LL** | |
| 7. Am proceeding in this direction | | | | 11. All well | |
| **N** | **Y** | **⌐L** | | **☐** | **⋮** |
| 13. No - negative | 14. Yes affirmative | 15. Not understood | | 17. Require compass and map | 18. Require signal lamp with batteries and radio |

## BODY SIGNALS

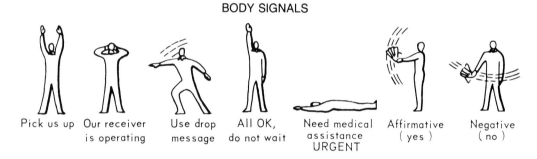

| Pick us up | Our receiver is operating | Use drop message | All OK, do not wait | Need medical assistance URGENT | Affirmative ( yes ) | Negative ( no ) |

## STANDARD AIRCRAFT ACKNOWLEDGEMENTS

**MESSAGE RECEIVED AND UNDERSTOOD**
Aircraft will indicate that ground signals have been seen and understood by —

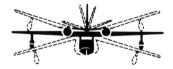

DAY OR MOONLIGHT
Rocking from side to side

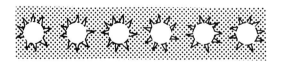

NIGHT    Making green flashes with signal lamp

**MESSAGE RECEIVED AND NOT UNDERSTOOD**
Aircraft will indicate that ground signals have been seen but not understood by —

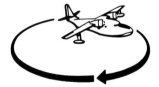

DAY OR MOONLIGHT
Making a complete right hand circle

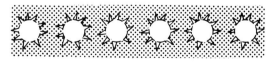

NIGHT    Making red flashes with signal lamp

During the day have damp material available to produce plenty of smoke, and try to vary the amount of smoke so that it does not appear to be naturally caused. By night flames will serve best to attract attention.

If possible, make signs on the beach or ground using stones, seaweed, soil or coloured materials. Attempt to make an SOS or MAYDAY sign, with letters as large as possible. Ideally each letter should be at least three metres in size.

## EXPLORATION

Depending on position, local conditions and the physical condition of surivivors, there may be good reasons for moving further afield. It is better if only two or three of the fittest survivors attempt any movement either inland or along the coast.

The direction taken should be marked so that return along the same route is possible.

Initially, it may be better to make for higher land to obtain an overall view. Look closely for signs of inhabitants, e.g. smoke, cultivated areas, electricity or telephone cables, pipelines, footpaths, roads, etc.

If signs of habitation are seen the fittest survivors should attempt to 'break out' to make contact. If no dwellings are visible, a possible alternative would be to break, tap or follow installations such as telephone or electrical cables, pipelines, navigational aids.

*Note:* Electrical cables may have high voltages and can be lethal.

## RESCUE

For survivors who have reached land there is a wider range of potential rescuers once the attention of the authorities has been attracted.

Rescue may come by sea in the form of small boats, or by air by helicopter. Rescue overland may be by road or across country by horse or on foot.

# APPENDIX A

## SIGNS OF DEATH

### Cessation of breathing

A mirror, such as a heliograph, held to the mouth and nose for several minutes is not dimmed by condensation from the person breathing.

### Cessation of circulation

The pulse at wrist or neck cannot be felt and the beating of the heart cannot be felt or heard. A string tightly tied around a finger will cause it to become bluish in life, but in death the finger will not change colour.

### Size of pupils

After death the pupils are large in size and do not decrease in size when a torch or bright sunlight is shone on the eyes.

### Coldness of body

The temperature of the body gradually falls to that of the surrounding air, beginning with hands and feet.

### Stiffening of body

This usually comes on three or four hours after death.

WARNING: SEVERE HYPOTHERMIA RESEMBLES DEATH!

## BURIAL AT SEA

Unless death occurs after contact with search aircraft or ships, any dead person should be buried at sea. To keep a body or bodies in survival craft is unhealthy and will badly affect morale. A record should be kept of any such burials.

Dead people should be stripped of any clothing which may be useful for warming the living.

Personal effects should be kept and handed to the appropriate authorities when rescued.

# APPENDIX B

## LIFEBOAT ENGINES

Starting and operating lifeboat engines varies between the different makes of engines. All seafarers should be familiar with the procedures for starting and operating the particular engines fitted to the lifeboats carried by the ships in which they serve.

Ships constructed after 1 July 1986 will be provided with water-resistant instructions for starting and operating the engine, which will be mounted near the engine controls. In general the following instructions apply to lifeboat engines.

### To start engine:

(1) Place gearbox in neutral.

(2) Check that fuel cock is open.

(3) Place fuel lever in 'start', or 'run' position or, if no specific positions are marked, to 1/2 speed setting.

(4) Set cold start or excess fuel device if fitted.

(5) If air cooled open vents.

(6) Hand start:

a  Lift decompressor lever(s).

b  Remove handle from stowage position and engage in starting slot.

c  Turn handle in direction of rotation as fast as possible then release decompressor lever(s). Keep turning the starting handle. The engine should now start.

d  Remove handle and return to stowage position.

e  If cold start device has been activated set lever to run position.

(7) Mechanical start:

a. Make sure the decompressor lever(s) is (are) not engaged.

b. Activate starter, release as soon as engine fires.

c. Do not operate electric starter motor for more than 20 seconds at a time.

d. If cold start device has been activated set lever to run position.

(8) Stopping engine:

Do *not* lift decompressor lever(s) to stop engine; use engine shut off device.

## WEEKLY INSPECTION

At weekly intervals all lifeboat and rescue boat engines shall be run ahead and astern for a period of not less than three minutes, provided the ambient temperature is above the minimum temperature required for starting.

### The weekly inspection should include the following:

(1) Check fuel level in tank and top up if required.

(2) Check oil level in sump and top up if required.

(3) Check oil level in reduction gear if applicable and top up if required.

(4) Check coolant level in header tank if applicable and top up if required.

(5) Start engine.

(6) Check oil pressure (if gauge fitted).

(7) Check for oil leaks.

(8) Check for fuel leaks.

(9) If the engine is water cooled, check circulation and for leaks.

# APPENDIX C

## GENERAL SURFACE CURRENT DISTRIBUTION

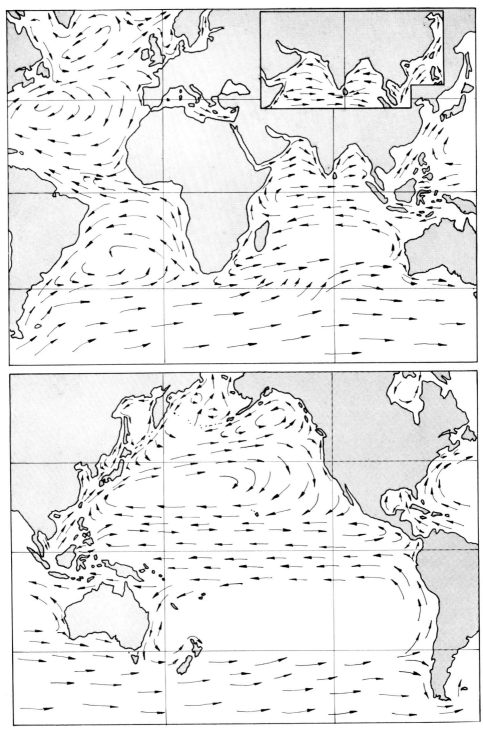

TOP — ATLANTIC AND INDIAN OCEANS
BELOW — PACIFIC AREA

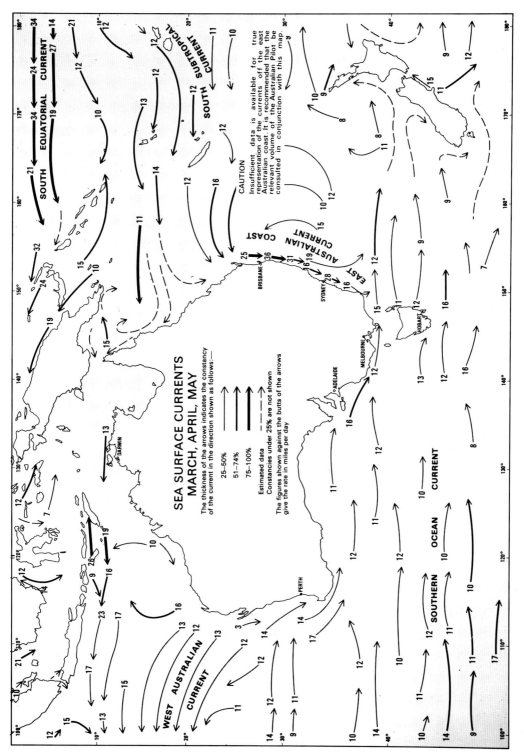

SEA SURFACE CURRENTS IN AUSTRALIAN WATERS
(i) MARCH APRIL MAY

85

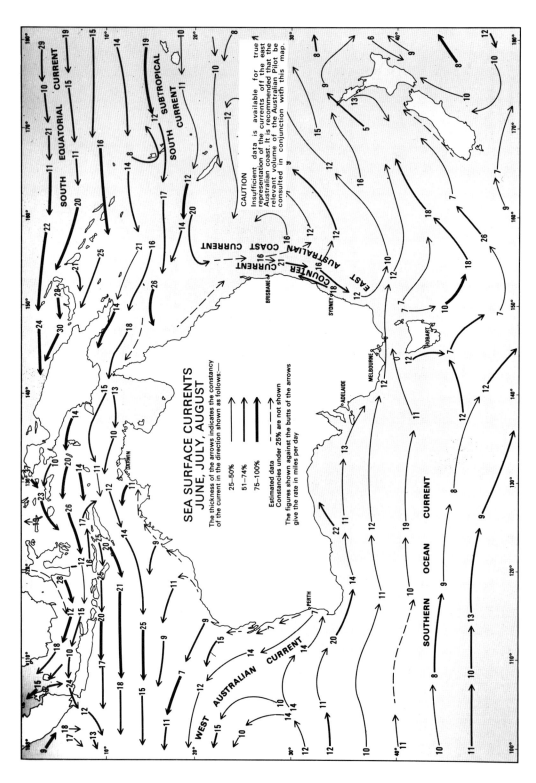

SEA SURFACE CURRENTS IN AUSTRALIAN WATERS
(ii) JUNE, JULY, AUGUST

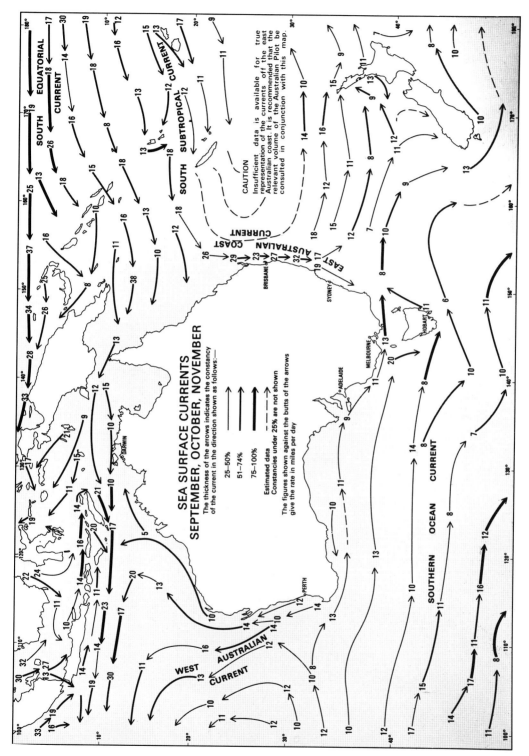

SEA SURFACE CURRENTS IN AUSTRALIAN WATERS

(iii) SEPTEMBER OCTOBER NOVEMBER

87

**SEA SURFACE CURRENTS DECEMBER, JANUARY, FEBRUARY**

The thickness of the arrows indicates the constancy of the current in the direction shown as follows:—

25–50%
51–74%
75–100%

Estimated data
Constancies under 25% are not shown

The figures shown against the butts of the arrows give the rate in miles per day

CAUTION

Insufficient data is available for true representation of the currents off the east Australian coast. It is recommended that the relevant volume of the Australian Pilot be consulted in conjunction with this map

SOUTH EQUATORIAL CURRENT

SOUTH SUBTROPICAL CURRENT

EAST AUSTRALIAN COAST CURRENT

WEST AUSTRALIAN CURRENT

SOUTHERN OCEAN CURRENT

DARWIN

PERTH

ADELAIDE

MELBOURNE

HOBART

SYDNEY

BRISBANE

**SEA SURFACE CURRENTS IN AUSTRALIAN WATERS**

(iv) DECEMBER JANUARY FEBRUARY

# INDEX

# Contents

# Sweet Options — what, when and where you use sugar

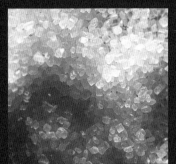

### Chelsea White Sugar — *reliable everyday*
Multi-purpose everyday sugar. The uniform size of the sugar crystals gives you a regular texture and consistency. The clarity of this pure-white crystal makes it the perfect ingredient for baking as it sweetens without affecting other flavours or the colour of the finished food or beverage. Use it on cereals, in tea/coffee/chocolate, as well as in baking, preserving and cooking.

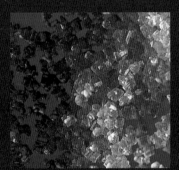

### Chelsea Raw Sugar — *everyday goodness*
Raw is the natural alternative to white. Full of natural goodness and energy, this caramel-coloured sugar is similar to white sugar in its broad range of everyday uses. Raw is used as a sweetener to enhance the flavour of coffee and in baking and cooking, where it improves the flavour and colour of the end result. As a topping, Raw sugar gives added crunchiness to porridge, fruit, desserts and muffins.

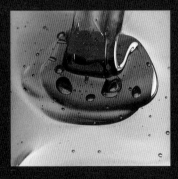

### Chelsea Golden Syrup — *gooey goodness, just pure fun!*
Drizzled over toast or pancakes, Chelsea original Golden Syrup is like a forgotten memory of what bliss truly is! The perfect baking ingredient for adding moisture, colour and flavour. Gingernuts, Brandy Snaps and Anzac biscuits are just a few examples of how Golden Syrup can be used to produce a deliciously rich, chewy result. Crumpets just wouldn't be crumpets without this uniquely flavoured topping either!

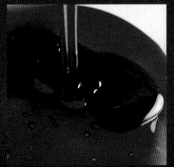

### Chelsea Treacle — *maximum flavour*
Ideal for creating dark, moist, flavoursome cakes and biscuits. Treacle has a richer deeper colour than golden syrup, and a stronger, slightly bitter flavour.

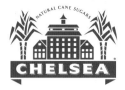

## Chelsea Caster Sugar — *the baker's sugar*

You can trust Chelsea Caster Sugar to give you the best baking result time after time. Very fine, evenly sized, white sugar crystals allow Caster Sugar to dissolve easily. This makes it ideal for pavlova, meringues, puddings, jellies and cake mixes. When used in baking, the smaller sugar crystals caramelise evenly so it produces a fine golden colour in the finished product.

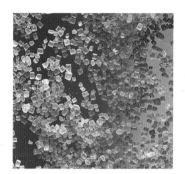

## Chelsea Icing Sugar — *celebrate with the best!*

Ahhh, the magical pleasure of silky-soft Icing Sugar, dusted over your favourite dessert to give it that mouth-watering finishing touch! This very sweet, finely powdered pure-white sugar is an essential pantry item. Chelsea Icing Sugar has a small amount of gluten-free starch to keep it free flowing and to prevent lumps forming, assuring you of the best quality every time. While no cake would be complete without decorative icing, Icing sugar can also be used to make goodies such as truffles, shortbread, cream fillings and marshmallow; anywhere a smooth, soft-finished texture is required. Icing Sugar also adds the perfect finishing touch when dusted over muffins, cakes or desserts.

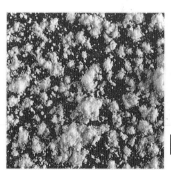

## Chelsea Soft Brown Sugar — *melts in your mouth!*

There is something mouth-watering about the caramel-fudge flavour and melt-in-the-mouth soft moistness of Chelsea Soft Brown Sugar. This ever-popular light-brown sugar is used in many recipes, both savoury and sweet. Its unique flavour makes it suitable for caramel, toppings, sauces and, of course, it is a Kiwi favourite on cereals, such as Weetbix and porridge!

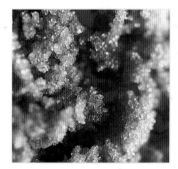

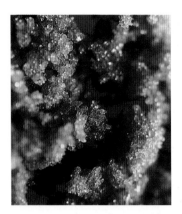

### Chelsea Dark Cane Sugar — *exotic enhancement*

This exotic sugar makes colour and flavour rich and full bodied. Dark Cane Sugar is a uniquely, moist dark-brown muscavado sugar. Its distinctive rich flavour comes from natural molasses cane syrup. Having a similar fine crystal size to Soft Brown Sugar, Dark Cane dissolves easily, making it ideal for sweetening fruits, puddings and fruitcakes, gingerbread or chocolate cakes. Create something very special by adding Dark Cane to your BBQ sauces, marinades, pickles and chutneys, chilli or curry. A small amount of Dark Cane Sugar is perfect to balance the hot, spicy flavours of Indian and Asian foods.

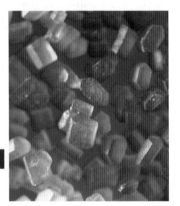

### Chelsea Coffee Sugar Crystals — *full-bodied flavour*

Why do things by halves? As the name suggests, Coffee Sugar is the right choice for coffee. The golden brown syrup left in this large crystal provides a unique flavour as the crystal slowly dissolves into your coffee, bringing out its full-flavour potential.

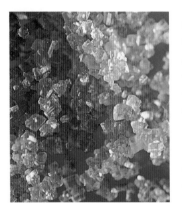

### Chelsea Demerara Sugar — *crème de la crème*

Demerara Sugar (pronounced Dem-err-rar-rar) is regarded by coffee connoisseurs as one of the finest sugars to enhance the flavour of coffee. It is only harvested from the canefields on the island of Mauritius in the Indian Ocean. It is derived from the initial pressing of the sugar cane, which allows some of the molasses syrup to remain in the crystal. This fine syrup adds a distinctive sticky molasses flavour and rich aroma. The clear-golden colour and distinctive crunch of these fine crystals give good colour to the crust of baking and toppings. Sometimes Demerara is referred to as 'turbinado' sugar in recipes.

# Cooking is Cool!

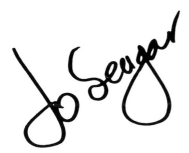

People love to get together to share food and it's really satisfying cooking something that everyone raves about.

Our recipes are easy to follow, with simple straight-forward instructions, which guarantee a fantastic success every time you make them.

We've covered recipes in here for all sorts of occasions: brunches; munchies; after-sport snacks; a big family lunch; impressive dinners; celebrations; birthdays; and even treats for a fundraising stall.

To be fit and healthy you need to eat a wide variety of foods from the four main food groups: cereals and breads (at least 5 servings a day); fruit and vegetables (at least 5 servings a day); milk and milk products (at least 2 servings a day); and lean meats (1–2 servings a day). A healthy balanced diet is all about eating enough to fuel growth, activity and appetite while enjoying but limiting treats and, of course, drinking lots of water — at least 8 glasses a day. So, come on you 'would be — could be' cooks, get that apron on, wash your hands and into that kitchen to get creative and have some fun. Let's get started!

Jo Seagar

## Weights & Measures
1 teaspoon (tsp) = 5 ml
1 tablespoon (tbs) = 15 ml
3 teaspoons = 1 tablespoon
1 cup = 250 ml

# Brunch

Boiled E

Panfried Eggs 'n

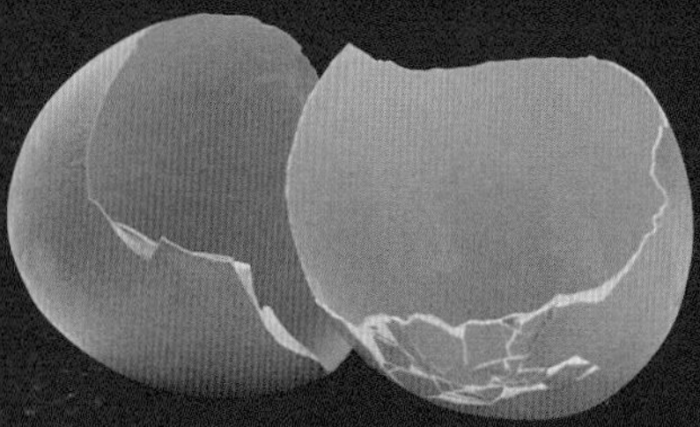

Scrambled E

Brunch in One 15

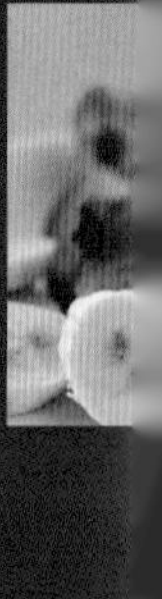

Warm Sugar-roas

Butterscotch Swirle

Stack 20 Go

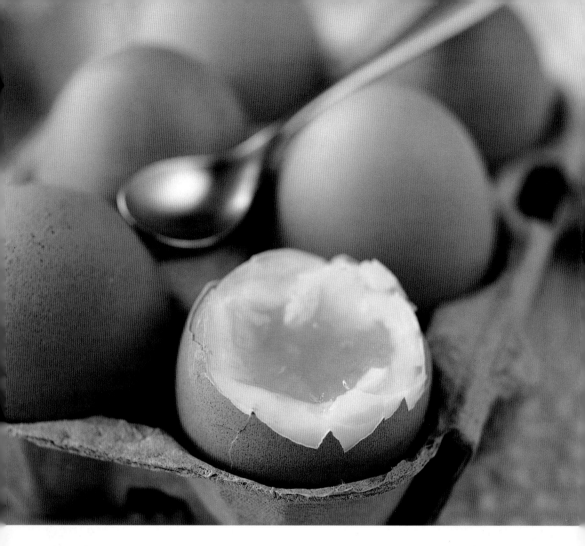

# Boiled Eggs

**PREPARATION TIME:**
½ A MINUTE
**COOKING TIME: 5 MINUTES**
**SERVES 4**

4 eggs

Place the eggs carefully in a small saucepan and cover with cold water. Bring the water to the boil over a high heat. As soon as the water boils, turn down the heat and simmer until the eggs are cooked to your preference:

- for runny, soft-boiled eggs: 3 minutes
- for firm whites but soft yolks: 5 minutes
- for hard-boiled eggs with very firm whites and a solid yolk: 10–15 minutes

Remove the saucepan from the heat. Take out the eggs using tongs, and place into egg cups.

Cut off each top, and serve with wholemeal toast cut into fingers. If you have made runny soft-boiled eggs, dip the fingers into the yolks.

# Creamy Eggs

**PREPARATION TIME: 3 MINUTES**
**COOKING TIME:**
**10–15 MINUTES**
**SERVES 4**

4 eggs

salt and freshly ground
  black pepper to taste

4 tablespoons milk or
  cream

4 tablespoons grated tasty
  cheese

toast to serve

Preheat the oven to 180°C. Spray 4 x 1 cup capacity ramekins with non-stick baking spray.

Break an egg into each ramekin. Season with salt and freshly ground black pepper. Spoon 1 tablespoon milk or cream over the eggs in each dish, then sprinkle with 1 tablespoon grated cheese.

Bake for 10–15 minutes until the eggs are set to your preference and the cheese has melted.

Serve in the ramekins with crisp toast.

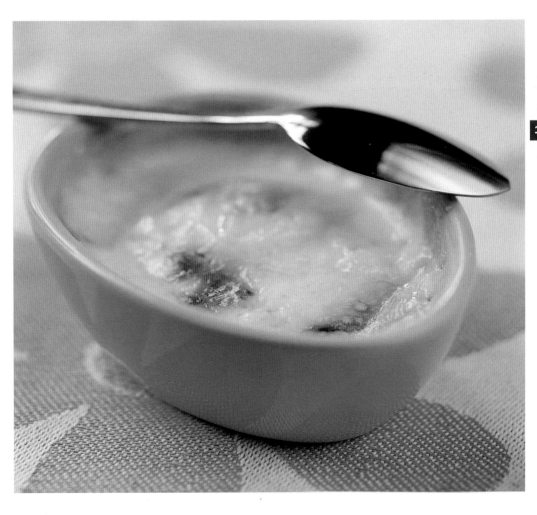

# Panfried Eggs 'n' Bread

**PREPARATION TIME: 5 MINUTES**
**COOKING TIME: 7–8 MINUTES**
**SERVES 2**

2 slices wholemeal toast-
  sliced bread

butter or margarine to
  spread

2 eggs

chopped fresh tomatoes or
  pan-fried mushrooms to
  serve (optional)

Preheat a frying pan over a medium heat.

Butter the bread on one side. Using a cookie cutter or small knife, cut out a shape, at least 4 cm x 4 cm, in the middle of each slice of bread. Have fun and use your imagination, the shape can be a heart, circle, your initials or animals, etc.

Place the bread slices and their cut-out shapes, buttered side down, in the heated frying pan. Once browned turn over and then carefully break an egg into each cut-out shape. Cook for 4–5 minutes until the bread is golden brown and the egg set.

Carefully spread some more butter or margarine on the top sides of the bread and shapes while they are cooking. Turn over and cook the second side for a minute or two and serve immediately.

These are great served with chopped fresh tomatoes or pan-fried mushrooms.

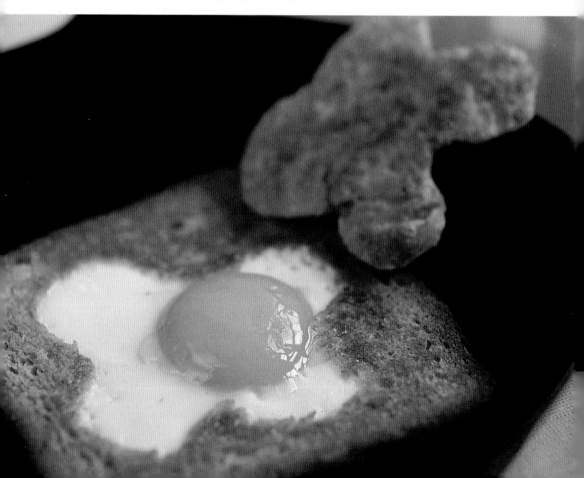

# Microwave Scrambled Eggs

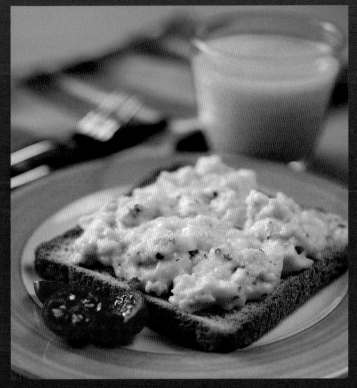

**PREPARATION TIME: 3 MINUTES**
**COOKING TIME: 3–4 MINUTES**
**SERVES 2**

4 eggs

½ cup milk

½ cup or small handful grated cheese (optional)

1 tablespoon chopped parsley

salt and freshly ground black pepper to taste

wholemeal toast to serve

Place the eggs in a medium-sized microwave-proof bowl or glass jug and whisk until frothy (a wire whisk is best for this job). Add milk and cook on high for 1 minute, then stir well. Cook for another 30 seconds on high and stir again. Add the cheese, if using, and parsley. Season with salt and freshly ground black pepper. Cook for about 30–40 seconds more. This will result in softly scrambled eggs. You may like them cooked a tiny bit more so they will perhaps need another 20–30 seconds on high.

Serve on wholemeal toast.

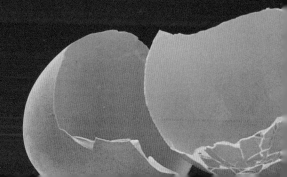

# Poached Eggs

**PREPARATION TIME: 2 MINUTES**
**COOKING TIME: 3 MINUTES**
**SERVES 2**

4 eggs

toast to serve

Half fill a small frying pan with cold water and bring to the boil. Turn the heat down until the water is simmering.

Add the eggs, one at a time, by first breaking them into a cup and then pouring them gently from the cup into the water.

Poach the eggs for 3 minutes, then carefully lift them out of the water with a slotted spoon, letting excess water drip off before serving on crisp toast.

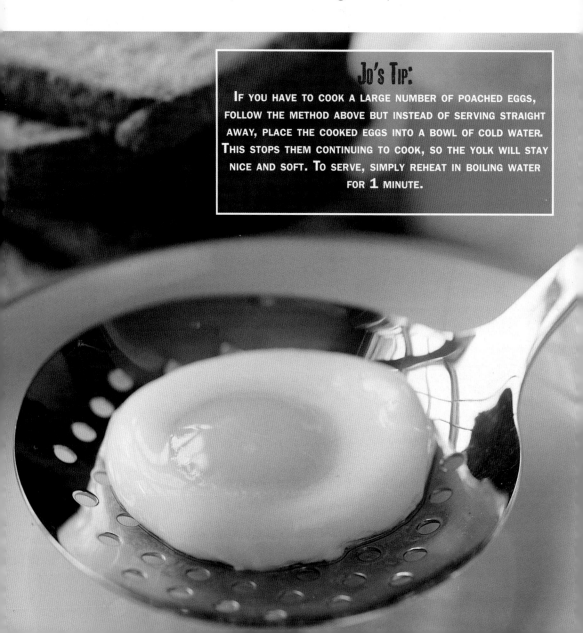

## Jo's Tip:

IF YOU HAVE TO COOK A LARGE NUMBER OF POACHED EGGS, FOLLOW THE METHOD ABOVE BUT INSTEAD OF SERVING STRAIGHT AWAY, PLACE THE COOKED EGGS INTO A BOWL OF COLD WATER. THIS STOPS THEM CONTINUING TO COOK, SO THE YOLK WILL STAY NICE AND SOFT. TO SERVE, SIMPLY REHEAT IN BOILING WATER FOR 1 MINUTE.

# Brunch in One

Cook the sausages in a non-stick ovenproof frying pan with the oil. Turn frequently and cook until they are browned and cooked right through — approximately 10 minutes. Drain the sausages on paper towels and cut into bite-sized pieces and wipe up any excess fat in the frying pan with paper towel.

Preheat oven to 200°C. Spray the frying pan with non-stick baking spray or oil.

Place the sausages and bread cubes in the frying pan. Beat the eggs and milk together and pour over the sausages and bread. Add the grated cheese, parsley and season to taste with salt and freshly ground black pepper. Stir gently to combine everything then bake in the oven for approximately 25–30 minutes until puffed up and golden brown. Cut into portions with a spatula or fish slice and serve.

**PREPARATION TIME: 10 MINUTES**
**COOKING TIME: 30 MINUTES**
**SERVES 4–6**

6 sausages

1 teaspoon oil

4 thick slices of bread, cut into 2 cm cubes, crusts on

6 eggs

½ cup low-fat milk

1 ½ cups grated tasty cheese

¼ cup chopped parsley

salt and freshly ground black pepper

Brunch

15

This is a fabulous breakfast, all cooked together. It is easy to serve and can be prepared the night before and kept in the fridge overnight all ready to cook in the morning. It is great to serve with tomatoes and mushrooms on the side.

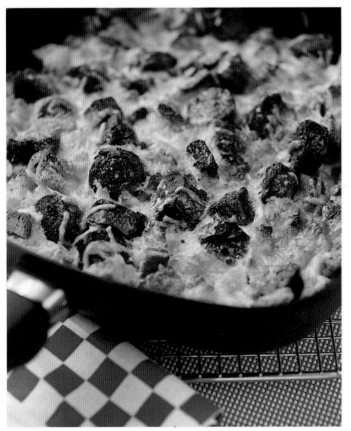

# Fab French Toast

In a food processor or blender, process the milk, sugar, eggs, vanilla, cinnamon and orange rind. Pour this mixture into a shallow, lasagne-type dish. Soak the slices of bread in the mixture.

Heat a large non-stick frying pan over a medium heat. Add the butter and oil and when this is hot and sizzling, add the soaked bread.

Fry both sides until golden brown. Drain on absorbent kitchen paper, then dust with icing sugar, if using.

Serve with crispy bacon and sliced bananas. Pour over golden syrup and, if you like, add yoghurt or whipped cream.

To cook crispy bacon: Allow at least 2 rashers of rindless streaky bacon per person.

- In a frying pan: spray a large non-stick frying pan with oil or non-stick baking spray and place over medium-high heat. Add the bacon and cook for 3–5 minutes, turning for even crispness. Drain on absorbent kitchen paper.
- In the microwave: place 3 pieces of absorbent kitchen paper on a microwave-proof tray or plate. Spread the bacon rashers on the paper and cook on high for 2 minutes. Turn the bacon over and continue to cook a further 2–3 minutes on high, watching carefully until it gets to just the right colour and crispness you prefer.

**PREPARATION TIME: 10 MINUTES**
**COOKING TIME: 15 MINUTES**
**SERVES 2–3**

This is a classic brunch or breakfast dish but also works well as a dessert without the bacon.

½ cup low-fat milk

½ cup Chelsea Caster Sugar

3 eggs

1 teaspoon vanilla essence

½ teaspoon ground cinnamon

finely grated rind of 1 orange

6–8 thick slices of diagonally cut French bread (day-old bread is best, or use toast-sliced wholemeal, white or raisin bread)

25 g butter or margarine

1 tablespoon oil

Chelsea Icing Sugar to dust

crispy bacon, sliced bananas, Chelsea Golden Syrup, yoghurt or whipped cream (optional) to serve

---

## Healthy Hint:

**Breads and cereals** — to keep energy levels high, eat at least five servings every day. If you are very active then you could need up to 10 or 12 servings a day — particularly guys.

Breads, pasta, rice and breakfast cereals are the carbohydrate foods and are an important source of energy and great to fill up on when hungry. And no, these foods don't make you fat. If you eat to your natural appetite (when your stomach tells you it's full) and limit fatty carbohydrate foods you won't get fat.

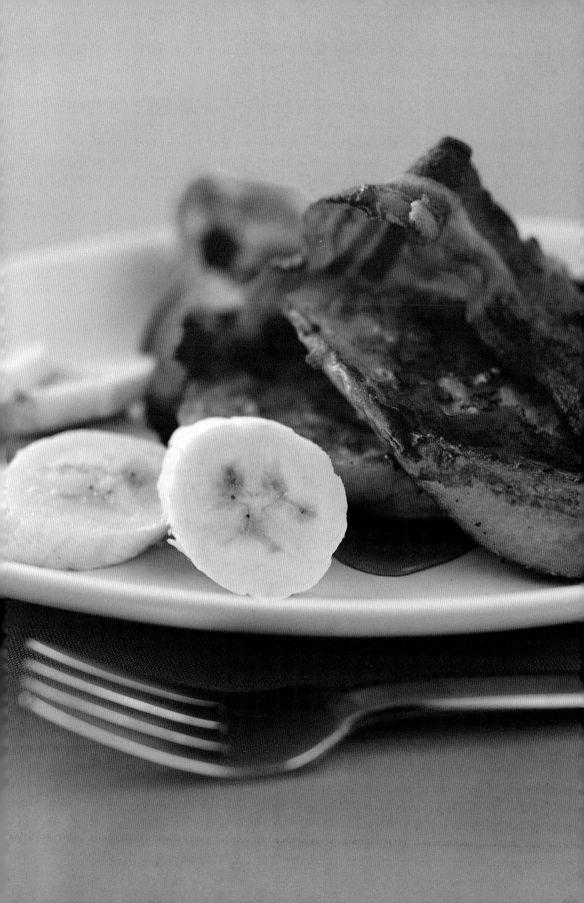

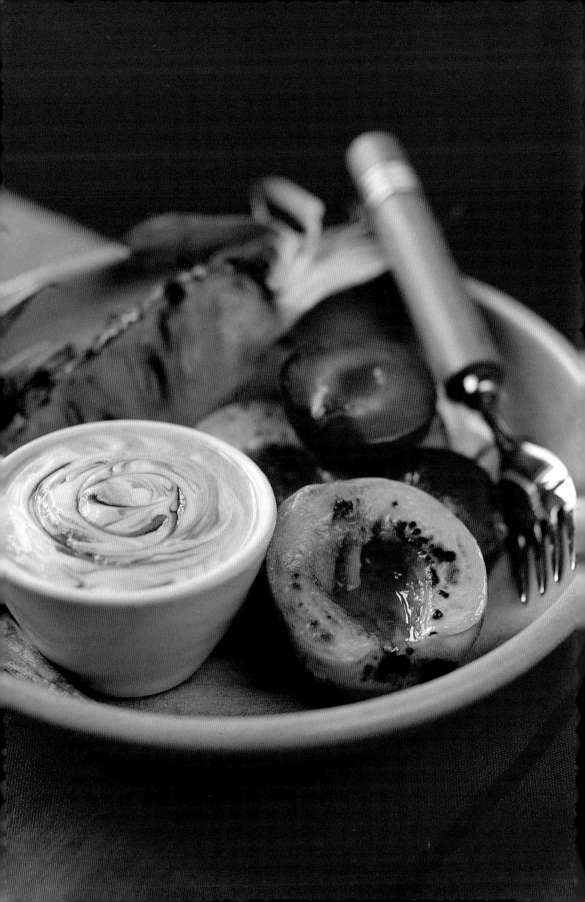

# Warm Sugar-roasted Fruit & Yoghurt

**PREPARATION TIME: 5 MINUTES**
**COOKING TIME: 5 MINUTES**
**SERVES 2–4**

2 plums, washed

2 peaches, washed

2 nectarines, washed

2 slices fresh pineapple

1 banana

2–3 tablespoons Chelsea
  Caster Sugar

fruit yoghurt to serve

Preheat the grill.

Cut the plums, peaches and nectarines in half and remove the stones. Cut the skin off the pineapple. Peel and slice the banana lengthways.

Place the fruit in a roasting dish and sprinkle with sugar. Place under the hot grill, and grill for about 5 minutes until the sugar is bubbling and has melted to a caramel–brown colour.

Serve the cooked fruit with thick fruity yoghurt, or Butterscotch Swirled Yoghurt (see below)

**Note:** You can also grill other fruits this way, such as pears, feijoas, persimmons, etc, depending on what is in season.

# Butterscotch Swirled Yoghurt

Place the yoghurt in a shallow dish. Sprinkle with sugar, then using a knife swirl the sugar loosely through the yoghurt. Don't completely mix in.

Cover the yoghurt and chill in the refrigerator for 1–2 hours. The sugar melts into the yoghurt and makes a lovely butterscotch-flavoured ripple or swirl through it.

Serve with fruit or cereal.

**PREPARATION TIME: 1 MINUTE,
PLUS 1–2 HOURS RESTING
TIME IN THE REFRIGERATOR
COOKING TIME: NO COOKING
REQUIRED
MAKES 2 CUPS**

2 cups thick natural yoghurt

1–2 tablespoons Chelsea
  Dark Cane Sugar

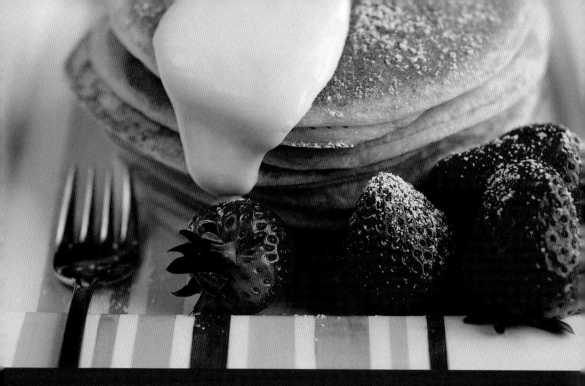

# Pancake Stack

**PREPARATION TIME: 5 MINUTES**

**COOKING TIME: 10–15 MINUTES**

**MAKES 10 PANCAKES**

1 ½ cups low-fat milk

4 tablespoons vegetable oil

3 eggs

1 teaspoon baking powder

1 ½ cups flour

Chelsea Golden Syrup, sliced bananas and crispy bacon, or strawberries and yoghurt to serve

Preheat a large non-stick frying pan or a non-stick electric frying pan on medium-high heat.

Place all the ingredients in a blender. Secure the lid firmly and process until smooth. Transfer the mixture to a jug that pours easily.

Wipe the surface of the heated frying pan with a few drops of oil on a paper towel.

Carefully pour about 3 tablespoons of the mixture into the pan. It should spread out to about the size of a saucer or small plate. Don't make the pancakes too big as they become difficult to turn. When the pancake surface is covered in bubbles, carefully turn it over and cook the other side.

Place the cooked pancake on absorbent kitchen paper, and keep covered with a tea towel while you cook the remainder of the batch.

Serve with golden syrup, sliced bananas and crispy bacon, or with strawberries and yoghurt.

## Variation:
Make the mixture as above but sprinkle some fresh blueberries, dried cranberries or raisins over the pancake mixture when you have just poured it in the pan. Turn and cook the second side as usual.

# Go For It! NRG Muffins

**PREPARATION TIME:**
**20** MINUTES
**COOKING TIME: 20** MINUTES
**MAKES 12**

2 cups flour

4 teaspoons baking powder

1 egg

¼ cup oil (vegetable, soya or canola)

1 ¼ cups low-fat milk

½ cup grated carrot

½ cup sultanas

½ cup grated, unpeeled apple

2 tablespoons coconut

¾ cup Chelsea Raw Sugar

1 teaspoon cinnamon

Chelsea Icing Sugar to dust (optional)

Preheat the oven to 200°C. Spray a tray of 12 muffin tins with non-stick baking spray or line each tin with a paper case.

Stir all the ingredients together until just combined. Spoon into the prepared muffin tins, and bake for 15–20 minutes until well risen and golden brown. Cool for 2–3 minutes in the muffin tins before gently twisting the muffins out to cool completely on a wire cake rack.

Dust with icing sugar if desired. These can be spread with butter or margarine if you like, or just eat them on the run.

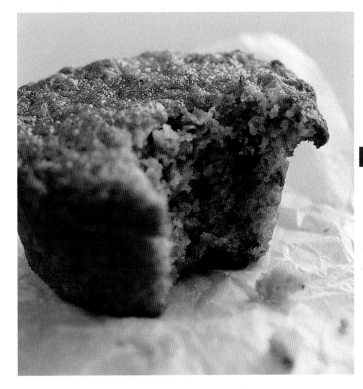

# Lunch

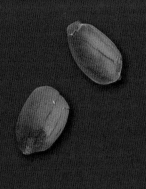

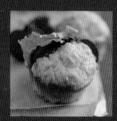

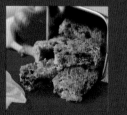

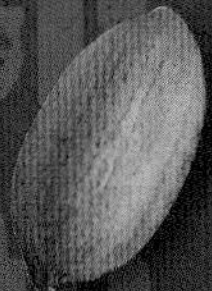

ut Crunch Biscuits 24

aisin Oaty Biscuits 24

Choc Chip Muffins 25

aiian Pizza Muffins 26

s 27 Mini Meatloaf 28

nchie Muesli Bars 29

conut Rough Slices 30

Chunk Oat Cookies 31

# Peanut Crunch Biscuits

**PREPARATION TIME:**
**10 MINUTES**
**COOKING TIME: 20 MINUTES**
**MAKES 24**

2 cups crunchy peanut
butter

2 cups Chelsea Caster
Sugar

2 eggs

Preheat the oven to 170°C. Line a baking tray with baking paper or spray with non-stick baking spray.

Mix all the ingredients together until well combined. Place teaspoonfuls of mixture on the prepared tray, leaving room for spreading. Using a wet fork, flatten the balls of mixture.

Bake for 16–20 minutes until golden brown. Carefully lift the biscuits off to cool completely on a wire cake rack.

Store in an airtight container when cold.

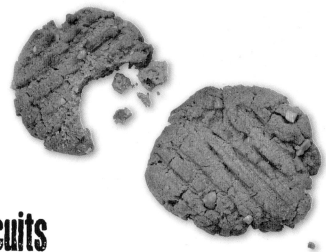

24

# Raisin Oaty Biscuits

**PREPARATION TIME:**
**10 MINUTES**
**COOKING TIME: 25 MINUTES**
**MAKES 40 BISCUITS**

1 cup Chelsea White Sugar

2 eggs

125 g butter

1 teaspoon vanilla essence

2 ½ cups rolled oats

2 ½ cups flour

1 cup seedless raisins or
sultanas

Preheat the oven to 180°C. Line two baking trays with baking paper or spray with non-stick baking spray.

Place sugar, eggs, butter and vanilla in a food processor and process until creamy.

Mix in the rolled oats and flour. Add the raisins and use the pulse button to quickly mix them in. Don't over process or you will chop up the raisins too much.

Place teaspoonfuls of the mixture on the prepared trays, allowing a little room between for spreading. Dip a fork in cold water and press the biscuits flat.

Bake for 20–25 minutes until golden brown. Cool on a wire cake rack.

Store in an airtight container.

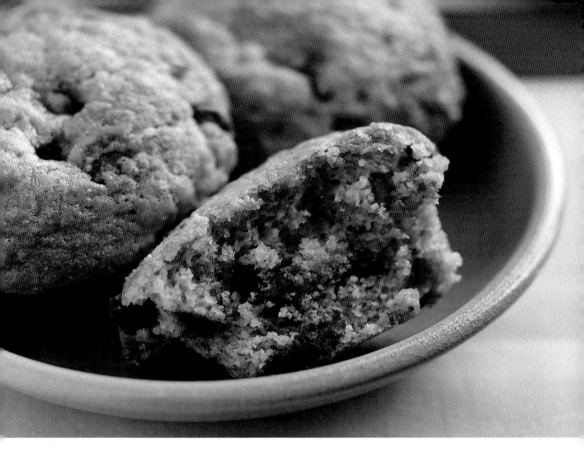

# Banana Choc Chip Muffins

Preheat the oven to 180°C. Spray a tray of 12 muffin tins with non-stick baking spray.

Place the eggs, bananas, oil, milk and sugar in a large bowl and beat together lightly. Mix in the flour, baking powder and chocolate chips. Don't overmix — the ingredients should just be gently stirred together to combine.

Spoon into the prepared tins and bake for 15–18 minutes until puffed and golden brown. Cool for 2 minutes in the tins then gently twist and ease the muffins out to cool on a wire cake rack.

## Jo's Tip:

ALWAYS SOAK THE MUFFIN TINS STRAIGHT AWAY AS SOON AS YOU'VE REMOVED THE MUFFINS. THIS MEANS THE TINS CLEAN UP EASILY AND YOU DON'T HAVE TO SCRUB AT THEM AND RISK RUINING THEIR LOVELY SHINY NON-STICK SURFACE.

**PREPARATION TIME: 8 MINUTES**
**COOKING TIME:**
**15–18 MINUTES**
**MAKES 12**

2 eggs

2 ripe bananas, peeled and mashed

¼ cup oil (vegetable, soya or canola)

1 cup low-fat milk

¾ cup Chelsea Soft Brown Sugar

2 ½ cups flour

4 teaspoons baking powder

1 cup chocolate chips

# Hawaiian Pizza Muffins

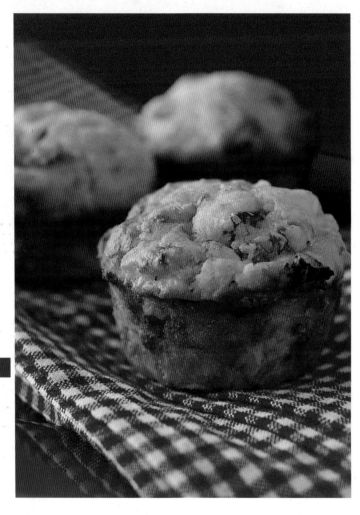

PREPARATION TIME: **8** MINUTES
COOKING TIME: **30** MINUTES
MAKES **12**

These combine all the flavours of everybody's favourite Hawaiian pizza in a convenient easy-to-eat muffin.

2 cups flour

4 teaspoons baking powder

1 ½ cups grated cheese

1 cup crushed pineapple in juice, drained (add ice and water and drink the juice)

½ teaspoon salt

4 rashers lean rindless bacon, chopped

2 tablespoons chopped parsley

¼ cup oil

1 egg

1 ¼ cups low-fat milk

Preheat the oven to 180°C. Spray a tray of 12 muffin tins with non-stick baking spray.

Place all ingredients in a large bowl and gently mix together until just combined. Don't overmix or the muffins will be rather heavy and solid — light muffins need a light mixing.

Spoon into the prepared muffin tins and bake for 25–30 minutes until puffed up and golden brown. Cool for 5 minutes in the tins then tip out to cool completely on a wire cake rack.

# Cheese Muffins

**PREPARATION TIME:**
**10–15 MINUTES**

**COOKING TIME: 20 MINUTES**

**MAKES 12**

2 cups flour

4 teaspoons baking powder

½ teaspoon salt

¼ cup oil

1 egg

1 ¼ cups milk

1 generous cup or a good handful of grated cheese

## Jo's Tip:

FOR A LOVELY SHINY CHEESY TOPPING, PLACE A FEW SHREDS OF GRATED CHEESE ON THE SURFACE OF EACH MUFFIN BEFORE BAKING. A FEW EXTRA TABLESPOONS WILL BE SUFFICIENT FOR THE **12** MUFFINS.

Preheat the oven to 200°C. Spray a tray of 12 muffin tins with non-stick baking spray.

Place all ingredients in a large bowl and gently mix together until just combined. Don't overwork the mixture or the muffins will be tough and chewy.

Spoon into the prepared muffin tins and bake for 15–20 minutes until golden brown. Cool muffins on a wire cake rack.

These can be eaten plain or filled like little bread rolls for a great lunch idea.

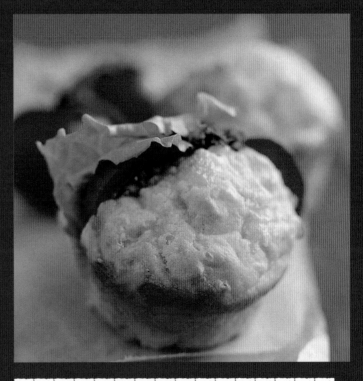

**Healthy Hint:** Fruits and vegetables — eat at least five servings a day. Fruits and vegetables are full of valuable vitamins and minerals that are important for good health and also aid in keeping your skin and hair healthy. Being low in calories and high in fibre they are filling without being fattening.

# Mini Meatloaf

**PREPARATION TIME:**
**10–15** MINUTES
**COOKING TIME:**
**35–40** MINUTES
**MAKES 12** MUFFIN-SIZED
MEATLOAVES

750 g lean minced beef or lamb

250 g sausage meat

1 cup fresh breadcrumbs (see note)

½ teaspoon salt and ¼ teaspoon pepper

1 cup spicy pasta sauce or tomato sauce

additional spicy pasta sauce or tomato sauce to serve

28

These meatloaves are not only delicious on their own for lunch, but are also great served in a bread roll or hamburger bun with salad and cheese slices.

Preheat the oven to 180°C. Spray a tray of 12 muffin tins with non-stick baking spray.

Wear plastic disposable gloves, or wash your hands thoroughly first, and use your hands to mix all the ingredients together.

Divide the mixture into 12 portions and press into the prepared muffin tins.

Bake for 35–40 minutes until nice and brown on top. Cool in the tins for 5 minutes then carefully lift out.

Serve with spicy pasta or tomato sauce.

**Note:** To make 1 cup of fresh breadcrumbs, whiz up 2 slices of toast-sliced bread in a food processor. Breadcrumbs can be frozen in small ziplock plastic bags and used from frozen. This is a good way of using up stale bread.

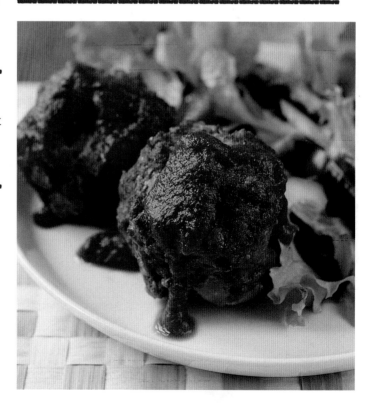

# Munchie Muesli Bars

PREPARATION TIME:
**15** MINUTES
COOKING TIME: **20** MINUTES
MAKES ABOUT **20** BARS

125 g butter or margarine

1 cup Chelsea White Sugar

2 tablespoons Chelsea Golden Syrup

1 cup flour

1 teaspoon baking powder

1 cup desiccated coconut

1 egg

1 cup mixed dried fruit (raisins, currants, dried cranberries, etc)

5 Weetbix or equivalent dry whole-wheat breakfast cereal, crushed

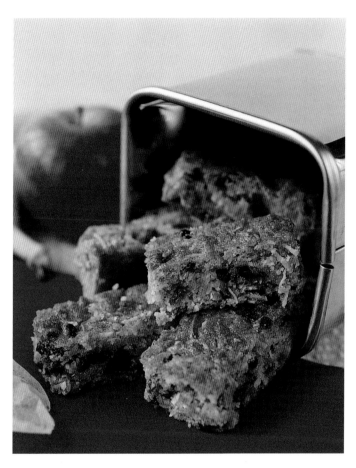

Lunch

29

Preheat the oven to 180°C. Spray a 20 cm x 30 cm sponge-roll tin with non-stick baking spray.

Place butter, sugar and golden syrup into a large saucepan, and stir over a medium heat until melted. Remove from heat, add all the other ingredients and mix thoroughly.

Press into the prepared tin and bake for 20 minutes. Cut into bars while still warm but leave in the tin until completely cold before removing.

Store in an airtight container.

# Coconut Rough Slices

PREPARATION TIME:
**15** MINUTES
COOKING TIME: **20** MINUTES
MAKES **28–30** PIECES

## Coconut rough slices

1 ½ cups self-raising flour

1 cup Chelsea White Sugar

1 ½ cups desiccated
coconut

3 tablespoons cocoa

200 g butter or margarine,
melted

## Chocolate icing

2 tablespoons hot water

25 g butter or margarine

2 cups Chelsea Icing Sugar

2 tablespoons cocoa

## Topping

2 tablespoons desiccated
coconut

Preheat the oven to 180°C. Spray a 20 cm x 30 cm sponge roll tin with non-stick baking spray.

Mix all the coconut rough ingredients together in a large bowl.

Press into the prepared tin and bake for 20 minutes. Cool in the tin while you make the icing.

To make the icing, place the water and butter in a microwave-proof jug or small bowl. Cook in the microwave on high for 30–40 seconds until the butter is melted. Beat in the icing sugar and cocoa until smooth, adding a little extra icing sugar if required.

Spread the icing over the coconut roughs while still warm and in the tin.

Sprinkle over the coconut and cut into slices, but leave to completely set and go cold in the tin before removing.

Store in an airtight container.

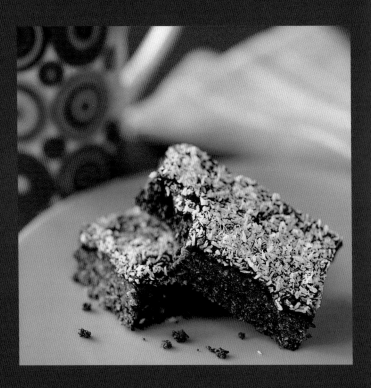

# Choc Chunk Oat Cookies

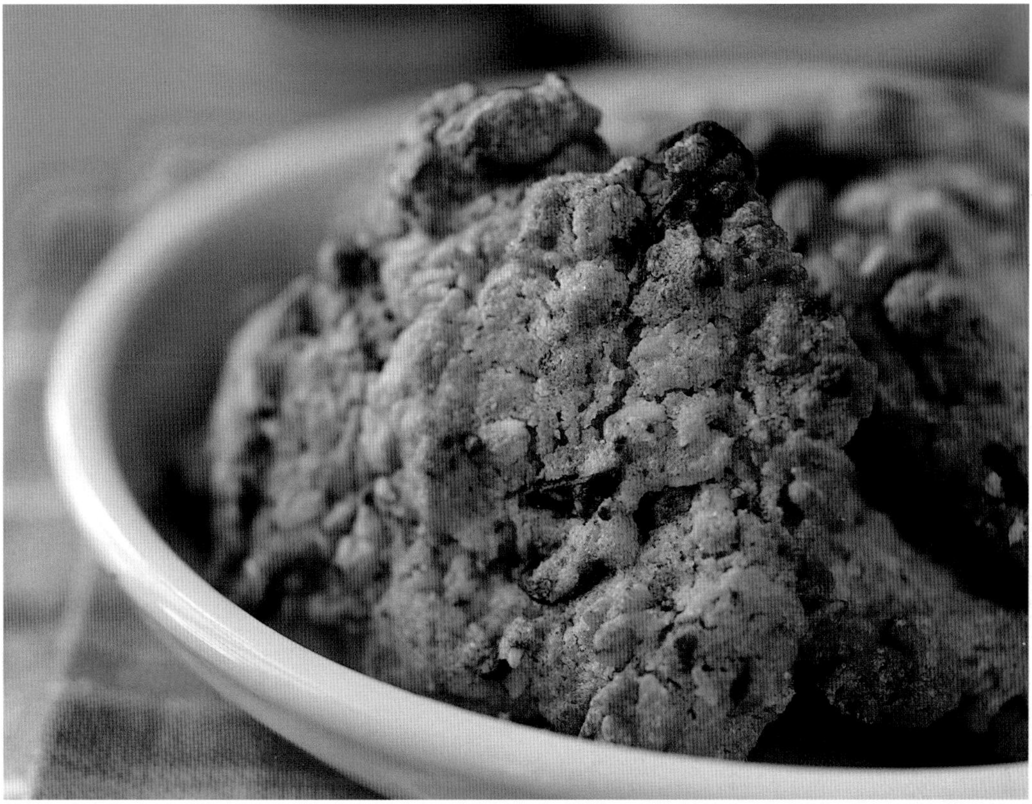

**PREPARATION TIME:**
**30 MINUTES**
**COOKING TIME: 20 MINUTES**
**MAKES 24**

250 g butter, softened

3 tablespoons sweetened
condensed milk

¾ cup Chelsea White Sugar

1 ½ cups flour

1 ½ cups rolled oats

1 teaspoon baking powder

200 g chocolate, roughly
chopped (milk, dark or
white chocolate, whatever
you prefer)

Preheat the oven to 180°C. Line two baking trays with
baking paper or spray with non-stick baking spray.

Beat butter, condensed milk and sugar together until
light and creamy. Add flour, rolled oats, baking powder and
chocolate chunks and mix well.

Place spoonfuls of the mixture on the prepared baking
trays, flatten and cook for 18–20 minutes until golden
brown. Cool on a wire cake rack.

Store in an airtight container.

# Snacks

# Choc Milk Ice Blocks

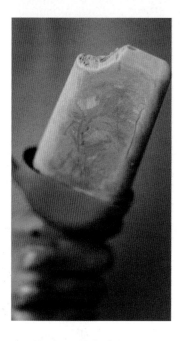

**PREPARATION TIME:**
**5 MINUTES, PLUS 12 HOURS**
**OVERNIGHT FREEZING TIME**
**COOKING TIME: NO COOKING**
**REQUIRED**
**MAKES 8 ICE BLOCKS**

1 teaspoon gelatine

½ cup cold water

¼ cup Chelsea Caster
Sugar

1 tablespoon cocoa

1 cup milk

½ cup full-cream milk
powder

1 teaspoon vanilla essence

Mix the gelatine and cold water in a microwave-proof small bowl. Leave for 3 minutes to set the gelatine.

Place the rest of the ingredients in a blender and mix well. Melt the gelatine by microwaving for 10–15 seconds on high, then pour into the blender with the cocoa mixture and blend until smoothly combined.

Pour into ice block moulds and freeze for at least 12 hours.

# Apple Spice Cupcakes

**PREPARATION TIME:**
**15 MINUTES**
**COOKING TIME: 25 MINUTES**
**MAKES 12**

¾ cup Chelsea Raw Sugar

1 cup wholemeal flour

1 cup flour

4 teaspoons baking powder

2 teaspoons mixed spice

1 egg

1 cup canned apple sauce,
stewed apple or apple
purée

¼ cup oil

¼ cup low-fat milk

½ cup sultanas

Preheat the oven to 180°C. Line a tray of 12 muffin tins with paper cases.

Mix all the ingredients together until just combined. Don't overmix or the cupcakes will be quite tough and solid. Spoon the mixture into the paper cases.

Bake for 20–25 minutes until lightly golden brown. Cool on a wire rack. Top with frosting (see page 94).

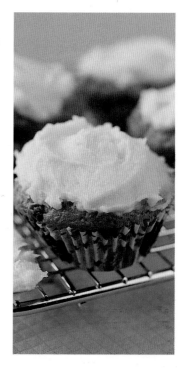

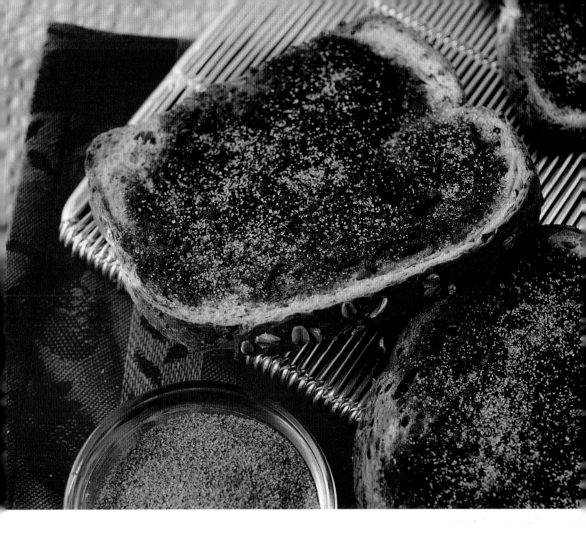

# Cinnamon Toast

**PREPARATION TIME: 4 MINUTES**
**COOKING TIME: 3 MINUTES**
**SERVES 2**

Preheat the oven grill. Place two slices of bread together and toast in a toaster (two slices in one slot) so that only one side of each slice is cooked. Lay the bread toasted side down on a baking tray.

Mix the margarine or butter, cinnamon and sugar together, and spread on the un-toasted side of each slice of bread.

Place under a hot grill for 2–3 minutes with the oven door open. Watch carefully as the bread toasts up crisply and golden and the cinnamon sugar mixture bubbles and melts. Carefully remove from the oven and don't forget to turn off the grill.

Cool for about 2 minutes then cut each piece of toast into 4 triangles and eat warm.

4 slices wholemeal bread

2 tablespoons margarine or soft butter

1 teaspoon ground cinnamon

3 tablespoons Chelsea Caster Sugar

# Honey Bubbles

**PREPARATION TIME: 4 MINUTES**
**COOKING TIME: ABOUT 8 MINUTES**
**MAKES 28–30 PIECES**

125 g butter or margarine

2 tablespoons honey

1 cup Chelsea White Sugar

2 cups rice bubble cereal

Spray a sponge roll tin, about 20 cm x 30 cm, with non-stick baking spray.

Place the butter, honey and sugar in a medium-sized saucepan. Stir over a medium-high heat until it boils. Turn down the heat, but keep the mixture just boiling for 5 minutes. Remove from heat and stir in the rice bubbles.

Press into the prepared sponge-roll tin and leave to set. Mark into squares when it is cool but not completely set.

When completely cold remove from the tin and cut along the marks. Store in an airtight container.

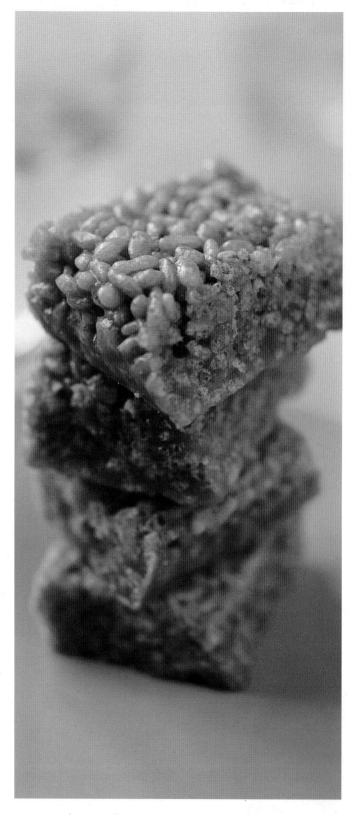

# Instant Pudding Biscuits

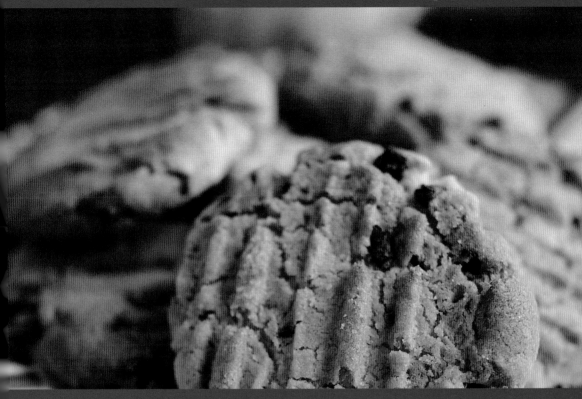

**PREPARATION TIME:**
**10** MINUTES

**COOKING TIME: 15** MINUTES

**MAKES 32**

150 g butter or margarine

¾ cup Chelsea White Sugar

1 egg

1 packet (70 g) instant
  pudding, any flavour,
  but our favourite is
  butterscotch

1 ½ cups flour

3 tablespoons cornflour

1 teaspoon baking powder

1 cup sultanas or chocolate
  chips

Preheat the oven to 180°C. Line a baking tray with baking paper.

Beat the butter and sugar together in a bowl. Add the egg, then the dry ingredients and sultanas or chocolate chips.

Roll into balls and flatten with a wet fork on the prepared tray. Make sure they do not touch each other and allow a little room for expansion. Bake for 15 minutes.

Cool on a wire cake rack and store in an airtight container.

**Healthy Hint:** **Make your snack a healthy one
— most of the time**

# Lemonade Scones

**PREPARATION TIME:**
**20 MINUTES**
**COOKING TIME: 20 MINUTES**
**MAKES 8–10 SCONES**

4 cups self-raising flour

300 ml cream

¼ cup Chelsea White Sugar

1 can (355 ml) lemonade

½ teaspoon salt

jam or honey to serve

Preheat the oven to 220°C. Cover a baking tray with a sheet of baking paper or spray well with non-stick baking spray.

Mix all the ingredients in a bowl to a smooth dough. Tip out onto a well-floured bench and cut into squares, or press out with a round cookie cutter.

Place the scones, just touching each other, on the prepared baking tray.

Bake for about 15–20 minutes until starting to turn pale golden. Check they are cooked through, and cool on a wire cake rack, covered with a clean tea towel (this keeps the scones lovely and soft).

Cut in half and spread with jam or honey when cool enough to eat.

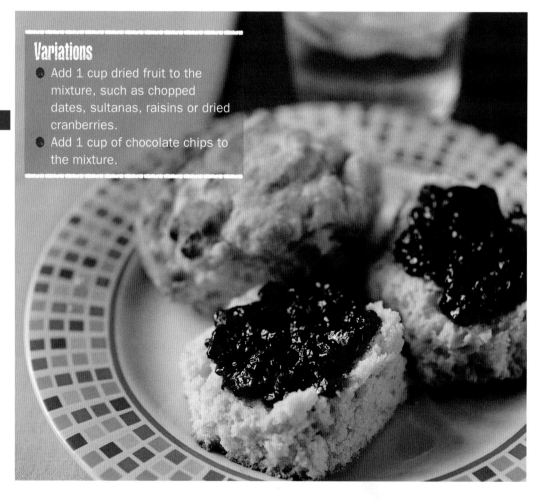

## Variations
- Add 1 cup dried fruit to the mixture, such as chopped dates, sultanas, raisins or dried cranberries.
- Add 1 cup of chocolate chips to the mixture.

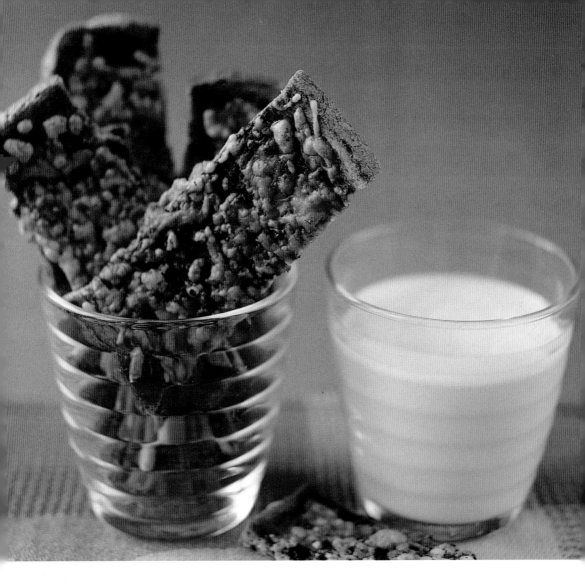

# Marmite or Vegemite Mousetraps

Preheat the oven to 160°C. Lay the bread slices on a baking tray and bake for about 8–10 minutes until dried and starting to crisp.

Remove from the oven and when cool enough to handle, spread the uncooked side lightly with Marmite or Vegemite and sprinkle with grated cheese. Cut each slice into 3 fingers and return to the oven to bake for a further 10 minutes until crispy, dry and golden brown.

Cool on a wire cake rack and store in an airtight container.

**Preparation time: 5 minutes**
**Cooking time: 20 minutes**
**Serves 2–4**

4 slices sandwich-sliced wholemeal bread

Marmite or Vegemite to spread

1 cup grated tasty cheese

# Mini Pizzas

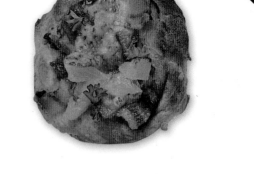

**PREPARATION TIME:**
**20** MINUTES
**COOKING TIME:**
**20** MINUTES
**MAKES 8** MINI
SAUCER-SIZED PIZZAS

These mini pizzas have a quick-to-make scone dough base.

### Pizza dough

2 cups self-raising flour

½ teaspoon salt

¾ cup low-fat milk

### Topping

2 tablespoons tomato sauce

1 ½ cups grated tasty cheese

4 rashers rindless streaky bacon

½ cup crushed pineapple, drained

2 tablespoons chopped parsley or chives

Preheat the oven to 220°C. Spray a baking tray with non-stick baking spray or cover it with a sheet of baking paper.

In a large bowl, mix all the pizza dough ingredients to form a soft dough.

With floured hands, break off 8 small balls of dough and press out, or roll out flat like little saucers. Place these on the prepared tray with room around them to spread out.

Spread tomato sauce over each base, just like buttering toast. Sprinkle over half of the grated cheese. Using scissors, cut the bacon rashers in half and snip each half into little pieces over the cheese. Divide the drained pineapple between the pizzas, then sprinkle with chopped parsley or chives and the remainder of the cheese.

Bake for about 20 minutes until puffed up and lightly golden brown on top. Cool for a minute or two then eat.

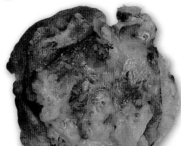

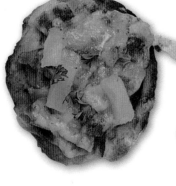

# Sweet or Savoury Pikelets

**PREPARATION TIME: 5 MINUTES**
**COOKING TIME:**
**20–25 MINUTES**
**MAKES 25 SMALL OR**
**12–15 LARGE PIKELETS**

½ teaspoon salt

1 teaspoon baking soda

1 cup low-fat milk

2 eggs

2 cups flour

½ cup Chelsea White Sugar

2 teaspoons cream of
   tartar

fruit jam or peanut butter
   to serve

To make Savoury Pikelets,
replace the sugar with
2 tablespoons of chopped
parsley or fresh herbs.
These are delicious served
with smoked salmon or
shaved ham and cream
cheese as finger food for
a party.

Place all the ingredients into a food processor or blender
and mix until smooth and well combined.

Heat a non-stick or electric frying pan over a medium
heat and lightly spray with non-stick baking spray.

Ladle teaspoonfuls of the mixture into the pan, allowing
plenty of room between them. It is best to cook just 2 or
3 pikelets at once. Cook for 2–2 ½ minutes per side, until
bubbles pop up on the surface. Carefully turn over and
cook the second side for another 2 minutes.

Cool on a wire cake rack. You only need to lightly oil
the pan once at the beginning, then just continue cooking
the remainder of the batch. Not oiling in between batches
gives the pikelets a lovely golden brown, even surface.

Serve with fruit jam or peanut butter.

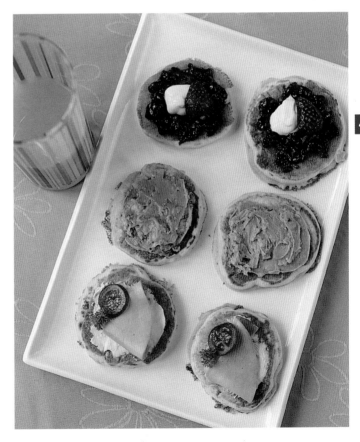

# Drinks Berry

## Frosty

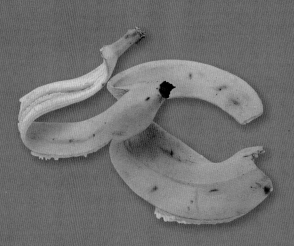 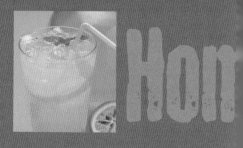 Hon

## Fruit Yoghurt S

## Chocolate wi

# Berrylicious Ice Cubes

**PREPARATION TIME: 5 MINUTES, PLUS OVERNIGHT FREEZING**
**COOKING TIME: NO COOKING REQUIRED**
**MAKES: 20 ICE CUBES**

12 blueberries

12 raspberries

12 small strawberries

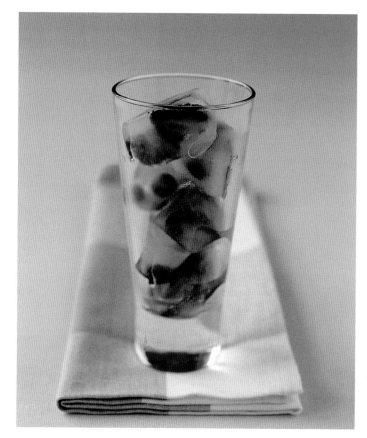

Place 3–4 of each variety of berry in each section of an ice cube tray. Fill with warm water (this makes really clear ice) and freeze overnight.

These ice cubes look great in party drinks.

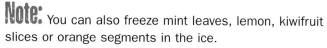

**Note:** You can also freeze mint leaves, lemon, kiwifruit slices or orange segments in the ice.

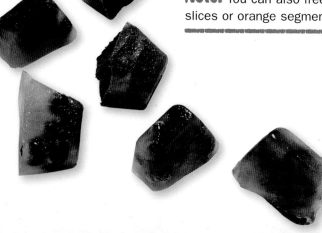

# Frosty Chocolate Shake

Place the milk, ice cream and chocolate sauce or ice-cream topping into a blender. Secure the lid firmly and process until thick and smooth.

Pour into a tall glass and garnish with chocolate sprinkles, if using. Grab a straw and go!

## Healthy Hint: **Milk and milk products,** such as cheeses, yoghurts and ice cream — eat at least two servings a day, preferably of low-fat options. These foods provide essential nutrients for growing bones, strong nails and teeth and are important sources of calcium and protein.

**PREPARATION TIME: 3 MINUTES**
**COOKING TIME: NO COOKING REQUIRED**
**SERVES 1**

1 cup low-fat milk

1 scoop ice cream

1 tablespoon chocolate sauce or ice-cream topping

chocolate sprinkles (optional)

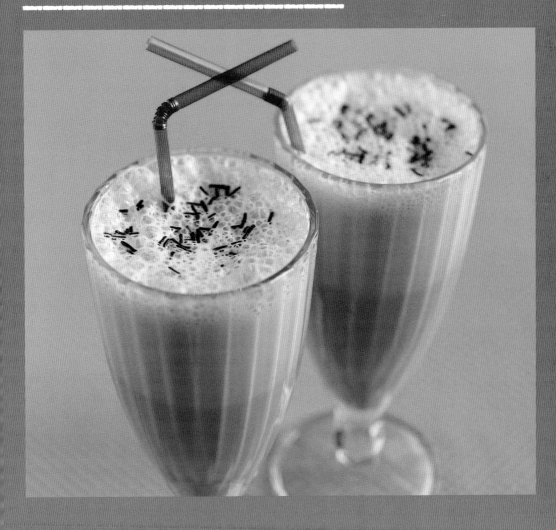

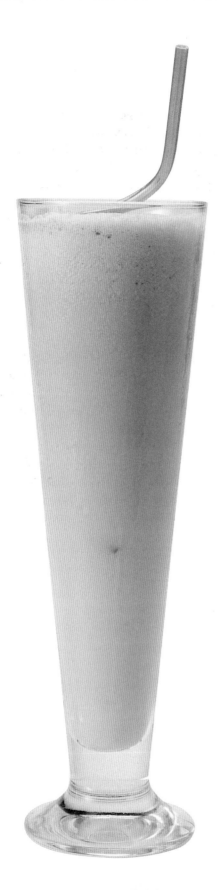

# Fruit Smoothies

**PREPARATION TIME: 3 MINUTES**
**COOKING TIME: NO COOKING REQUIRED**
**SERVES 2**

## Banana Strawberry Smoothie

1 ripe banana, peeled

6 strawberries, leaves and stalk removed

2 cups low-fat milk

2 scoops low-fat ice cream or frozen yoghurt

fresh fruit and mint sprigs to garnish

Place all the ingredients, except the garnish, in a blender. Secure the lid firmly and process until the mixture is thick and smooth. Pour into 2 big glasses, and decorate with pieces of fresh fruit and mint sprigs.

Drink with a thickshake straw — you'll probably need a spoon as well.

**Note:** You can invent your own flavoured smoothies by adding different fruits — apricots and peaches are great, so are mixed berries, pawpaw and passionfruit. Canned fruit in light syrup or fruit juice is also really good.

# Homemade Lemonade

Peel the rind off 2 lemons, taking care to get just the outer skin, no white pith (use a potato peeler for this).

Place the peel and 2 cups of the sugar in the food processor and run the processor until the rind is really ground up and the sugar is yellow and oily looking. Tip into a large saucepan.

Squeeze all 6 lemons and, to remove any pips, strain the juice into the lemon sugar mixture in the saucepan, add the remaining sugar and the citric acid. Place the saucepan on a medium heat and add the 3 litres of water, stirring until the sugar dissolves.

Cool, then pour into clean bottles and store in the refrigerator.

To serve, dilute with water: 1 part cordial to 3–4 parts water. To make fizzy lemonade, dilute with sparkling mineral water or soda water.

**PREPARATION TIME: 20 MINUTES**
**COOKING TIME: 5 MINUTES**
**MAKES 3 LITRES OF CONCENTRATED CORDIAL**

6 lemons, scrubbed in cold water

1 ½ kg Chelsea White Sugar

50 g (½ packet) citric acid

3 litres water

For a party, make pink lemonade by adding a few drops of pink food colouring to the cordial. Dress up the glasses with fancy straws, ice cubes (see page 44), slices of fruit and cocktail umbrellas or little plastic toys.

Drinks

47

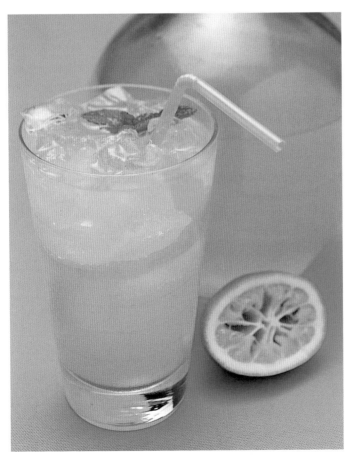

# Fruit Ju Slushies

**PREPARATION TIME:**
**2 MINUTES, PLUS 4 HOURS**
**FREEZING TIME**
**COOKING TIME: NO COOKING**
**REQUIRED**
**SERVES 2**

4 cups fruit juice (orange, apple & orange, etc)

2 tablespoons jelly crystals

Place the ingredients in a blender. Secure the lid firmly and process until well mixed. Pour into an ice cube tray and freeze until really solid — at least 4 hours.

Once frozen, place the ice cubes in a blender and process until slushy and liquid.

Pour into 2 big glasses and serve immediately with spoons and thick straws.

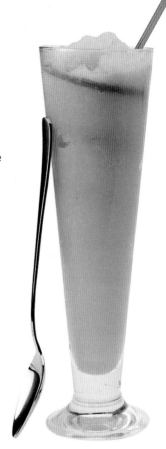

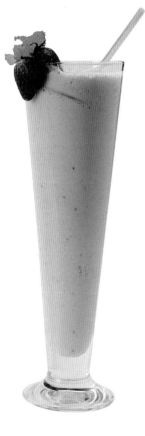

# Fruit Yoghurt Shake

**PREPARATION TIME: 3 MINUTES**
**COOKING TIME: NO COOKING**
**REQUIRED**
**SERVES 1**

1 cup fruit yoghurt

1 cup fruit juice (apple, orange, mango, etc)

1 cup ice cubes

Place all the ingredients into a blender. Secure the lid firmly and process until the ice is all crushed and the mixture is nice and smooth.

Pour into a big glass and eat with a combination of a straw and a spoon.

**Note:** If you only have plain yoghurt you can add half a banana or a tablespoon of jam to flavour the shake.

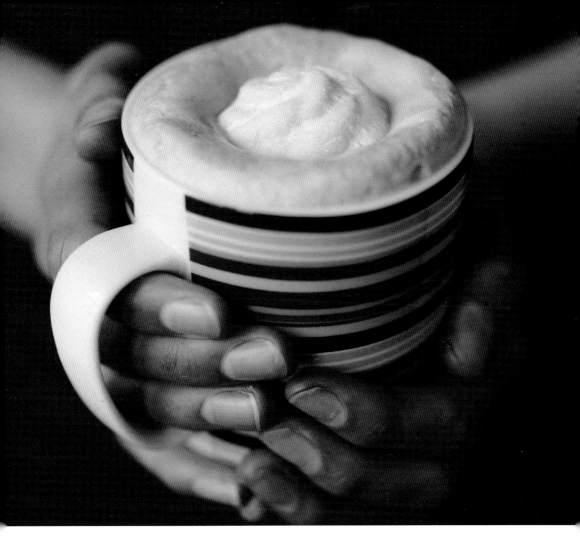

# Steamy Hot Chocolate with Marshmallows

**PREPARATION TIME: 2 MINUTES**
**COOKING TIME: 3–4 MINUTES**
**SERVES 2**

2 cups low-fat milk

1 tablespoon cocoa

1 tablespoon Chelsea White Sugar

½ teaspoon vanilla essence

2 marshmallows (optional)

Place the milk, cocoa, sugar and vanilla in a microwave-proof jug and whisk. Don't worry if it's not a very smooth mixture. Microwave on high power for 1 minute, then carefully whisk again. Cook for another 1 minute on high. Give the mixture a good whisk, but be careful as it is getting quite hot by now. Cook for a further 1–2 minutes until it is nice and hot and the sugar is well dissolved.

Pour into 2 mugs and float a marshmallow, if using, on the top.

# Dinner

Butter Ch

Baked Potatoes 54 Ques

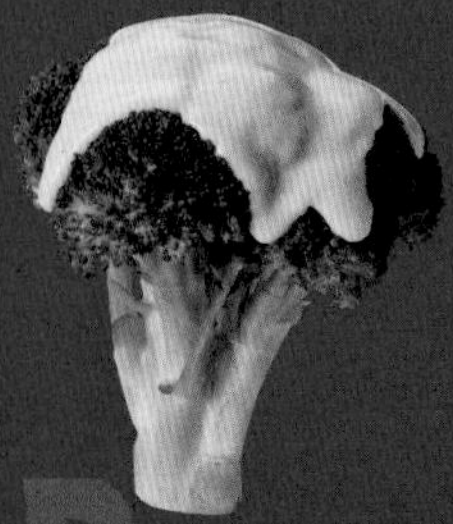

Crunchy Peanut Sa

Peach Salad 58 Spiced V

Macaroni Cheese 61 Gar

Carrots 64 Cheese Sau

Lemon Fish & Rice 68 N

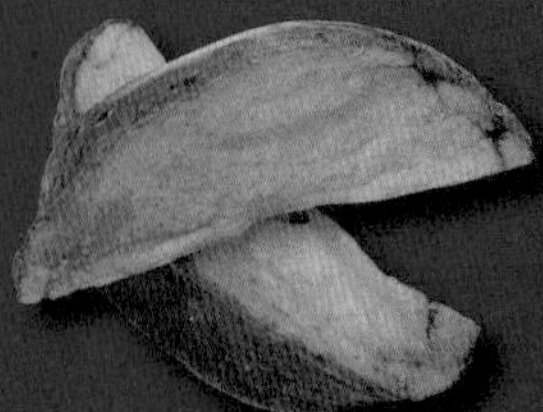

Sour Pork Stir

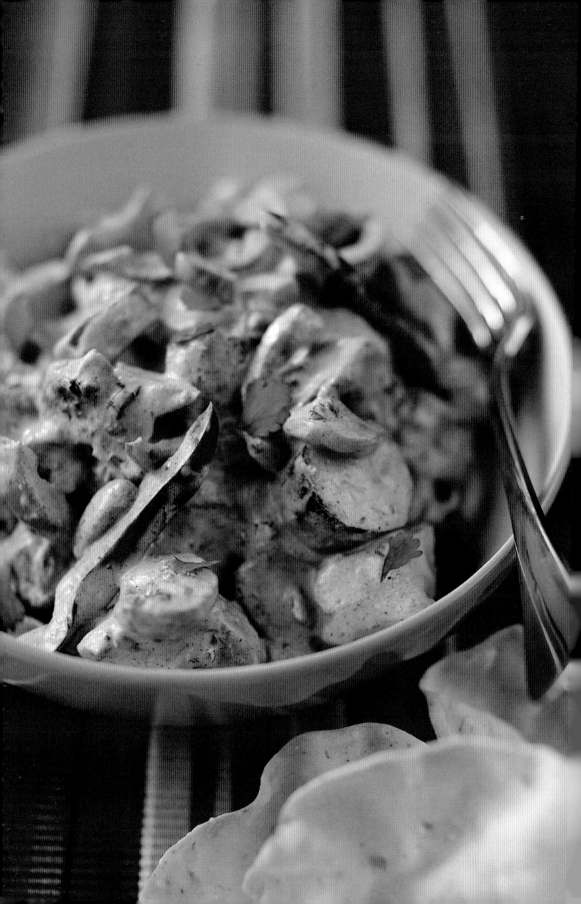

# Butter Chicken with Rice & Poppadoms

**PREPARATION TIME:**
**30 MINUTES, PLUS 3 HOURS**
MARINATING
**COOKING TIME: 40 MINUTES**
**SERVES 4**

## Butter chicken

4 skinless, boneless
  chicken breasts

3 tablespoons tandoori
  paste from a jar

1 tablespoon Chelsea Dark
  Cane Sugar

1 tablespoon oil

5 spring onions, chopped

3 cups button mushrooms,
  sliced

4 courgettes, cut into
  chunky slices

1 red capsicum, deseeded
  and sliced

¼ cup chopped parsley

¼ cup chopped coriander,
  including stalks and
  leaves

2 cups sour cream or thick
  yoghurt

extra coriander leaves
  to garnish

## Rice & Poppadoms

1 teaspoon salt

2 cups long-grain rice

8 small or 4 large
  poppadoms

Cut up the chicken breasts into bite-sized pieces and place in a small ovenproof lasagne or casserole dish. Spoon in the tandoori paste, sugar and oil and mix well to evenly coat the chicken. Cover with plastic food wrap and set aside in the refrigerator to marinate for 2–3 hours or preferably overnight.

Preheat the oven to 200°C.

Add the spring onions, mushrooms, courgettes, capsicum, parsley and coriander to the marinated chicken and stir to mix through. Bake for 35–40 minutes, stirring every now and then so the chicken cooks evenly.

When the chicken is halfway through cooking, prepare the rice and poppadoms.

To cook the rice, half fill a large saucepan with water. Add the salt and bring to the boil. Add the rice and boil for 12 minutes, stirring once or twice to prevent sticking. Drain the rice through a sieve.

To cook the poppadoms, place 1 poppadom at a time on absorbent kitchen paper in the microwave. Cook on high for 50–60 seconds or follow instructions on packet until puffed and crisp. Cool on a wire cake rack as you cook the remainder of the poppadoms.

Remove the chicken from the oven and stir in the sour cream or yoghurt. Sprinkle with coriander leaves.

Serve the butter chicken on the rice with a side serving of poppadoms.

**Healthy Hint:** **Lean meats** (such as beef and lamb), fish and chicken, dried beans, peas and lentils — one to two servings a day. These provide an important source of iron and protein and many other valuable nutrients that your body needs: lots of iron for growth, mental and physical activity and sports.

# Bubble 'n' squeak Baked Potatoes

PREPARATION TIME:
**15** MINUTES
COOKING TIME:
**30–60** MINUTES
SERVES **4**

4 medium-large potatoes, scrubbed but not peeled

2 tablespoons oil

3 rashers lean bacon, chopped

1 onion, peeled and finely chopped

2 cups finely shredded cabbage

3 tablespoons parsley, chopped

salt and freshly ground black pepper to taste

½ cup grated tasty cheese

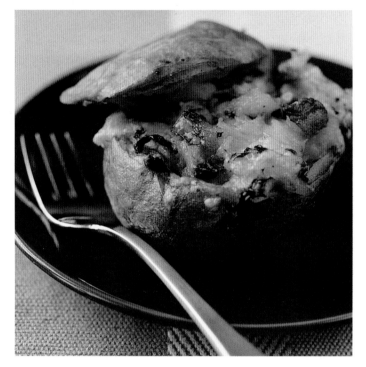

If using an oven, preheat to 200°C.

Bake the potatoes either in an oven for 30–40 minutes or in a microwave for 10–14 minutes, turning halfway through (halve the time if you use only 2 potatoes). They are cooked when they give when pressed. Remove them from the oven and allow to cool so that you can handle them comfortably. The microwaved potatoes will continue to cook during this standing time for 3–4 minutes.

Cut off the tops and scoop out the cooked potato into a bowl. Mash this potato with a fork.

Heat the oil in a large frying pan. Add the bacon and onion and cook for 3 minutes before adding the cabbage. Stir-fry for a few minutes. Add the mashed potato and parsley, and season with salt and freshly ground black pepper.

Spoon the mixture back into the potato jackets, sprinkle with grated cheese and replace the 'lids'.

Reheat the potatoes before serving. These can be prepared up to a day in advance and stored in the refrigerator.

# Cheesy Avocado Quesadillas

Lay out 4 tortillas.

In a small bowl, mix the spring onions, avocado, lime or lemon juice, chilli sauce and coriander or parsley. Spread this mixture over the tortillas as if you were buttering bread. Season with salt and freshly ground black pepper. Sprinkle over cheese and cover each one with another tortilla.

Heat oil in a large, preferably non-stick, frying pan. Add a tortilla sandwich and fry for 2 minutes each side. Keep warm in the oven while you cook the remainder, oiling the pan lightly between each one.

Cut into wedges to serve — this is easily done with kitchen scissors.

Quesadillas are Mexican sandwiches made with soft flour tortillas. They are super quick to make and are a neat change from the usual toasted sandwich.

8 soft flour tortillas

2 spring onions, chopped

1 firm but ripe avocado, peeled, stoned and chopped

juice of 1 small lime or ½ a lemon

2 tablespoons mild sweet chilli sauce

2 tablespoons chopped coriander or parsley

salt and freshly ground black pepper to taste

1 cup grated tasty cheese

1 teaspoon oil

Dinner

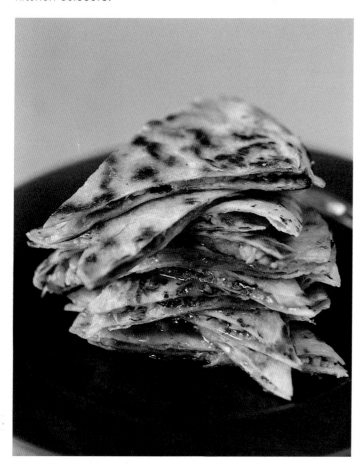

# Chicken Satay
## with Crunchy Peanut Sauce

Soak the satay skewers in water for at least an hour to prevent them from burning on the barbecue or under the grill.

Cut the chicken into long strips like fingers. You should aim to get 5 strips from each chicken breast.

In a shallow dish or plastic container, whisk the soy sauce, oil and garlic together. Add the chicken strips and stir to coat well. Cover the dish and set aside to marinate in the refrigerator for at least 3 hours or overnight.

Thread the chicken strips onto the soaked bamboo skewers, in and out as if you are sewing.

Cook the satays on a barbecue hot plate or under the grill, turning until they are cooked evenly and dark golden brown. Serve the satays with Crunchy Peanut Sauce.

**PREPARATION TIME:**
**10 MINUTES, PLUS 3 HOURS MARINATING**
**COOKING TIME: 10 MINUTES**
**MAKES 20 SATAYS**

### Satays

20 bamboo satay skewers

4 skinless, boneless chicken breasts

¼ cup soy sauce

¼ cup oil

2–3 cloves of garlic, crushed

# Crunchy Peanut Sauce

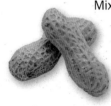

Mix all the ingredients together in a small bowl. If you want the sauce thinner, add a little milk. Taste the sauce and add salt and freshly ground black pepper, or extra sweet chilli sauce to season.

**PREPARATION TIME: 5 MINUTES**
**COOKING TIME: NO COOKING REQUIRED**
**MAKES 2 CUPS**

1 cup crunchy peanut butter

2 tablespoons sweet chilli sauce

1 cup low-fat sour cream or thick natural unsweetened yoghurt

2 tablespoons chopped parsley

salt and freshly ground black pepper to taste

## Jo's Tip:
You can add other items to the skewers to turn them into kebabs. Red and green capsicums, baby mushrooms, cherry tomatoes, pineapple, etc.

# Crunchy Spiced Wedges

Preheat the oven to 200°C.

Cut the potatoes in half lengthways, then cut each half into wedges.

Place the oil, garlic salt and paprika into a large ziplock plastic bag. Add the potato wedges and seal the bag. Shake and squish the bag around so that the wedges get well coated.

Place the wedges in a single layer in an oven roasting dish. Bake for about 35–40 minutes. Stir them once or twice during cooking.

Serve with tomato or sweet chilli sauce or for a treat try sour cream or yoghurt.

**PREPARATION TIME: 5 MINUTES**
**COOKING TIME: 40 MINUTES**
**SERVES 2–4**

4 large potatoes, skin on, well scrubbed and dried

1 tablespoon oil

1 teaspoon garlic salt

1 teaspoon paprika

tomato or sweet chilli sauce, or sour cream or yoghurt to serve

## Jo's Tip:
Kumara, parsnips and pumpkin can all be cooked the same way. Peel them first though, as their skins can be very tough.

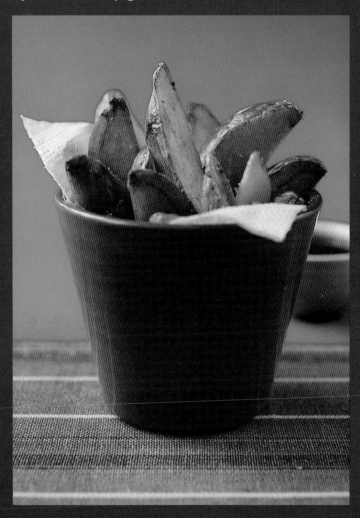

# Fab Corn Fritters

**PREPARATION TIME:**
**10** MINUTES
**COOKING TIME: 30** MINUTES
**MAKES 8–10** GOOD-SIZED
FRITTERS OR **20** LITTLE
FINGER-FOOD ONES

1 x 410 g can cream-style
  sweetcorn

1 cup self-raising flour

¼ cup low-fat milk

3 eggs, separated

salt and freshly ground
  black pepper to taste

2 tablespoons chopped
  parsley

5 tablespoons oil, to cook

chilli sauce, tomato sauce
  or salsa to serve

Also great for lunch, or
make little fritters to serve
as a finger-food snack.

In a large bowl, mix together the sweetcorn, flour, milk, egg yolks, salt and freshly ground black pepper and parsley. In a separate bowl, beat the egg whites until stiff and fluffy. Fold these gently into the corn mixture.

Heat the oil in a large non-stick frying pan over a medium-high heat. Cook spoonfuls of the mixture for about 3 minutes each side, or until puffed up and golden brown.

Drain on absorbent kitchen paper and keep warm in the oven while you cook the remainder of the batch.

Serve with chilli sauce, tomato sauce or salsa.

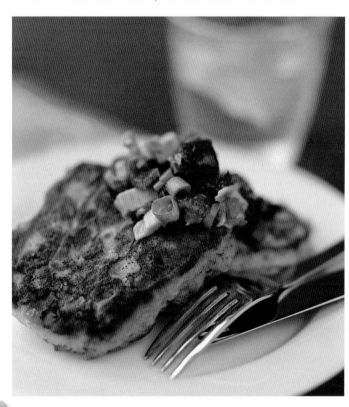

# Macaroni Cheese: Comfort Food at its Best!

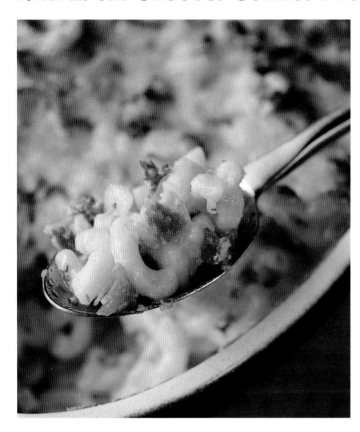

**PREPARATION TIME:**
**10** MINUTES
**COOKING TIME:**
**20–25** MINUTES
**SERVES 3–4**

1 ½ cups dried macaroni pasta

1 teaspoon mild mustard (optional)

2 cups low-fat milk

salt and freshly ground black pepper to taste

3 tablespoons cornflour

2 rashers rindless bacon, finely chopped

1 small onion, peeled and finely chopped

2 cups grated tasty cheese

1 tablespoon chopped parsley to serve

2 tomatoes, chopped, to serve

Dinner

61

Cook the pasta in a large saucepan of gently boiling, salted water until tender (al dente), about 7–8 minutes, but check on the macaroni packet for instructions.

While the pasta is cooking, spray an oven-proof pie or small lasagne dish, about 20 cm x 20 cm, with non-stick baking spray. Preheat the oven grill to medium high.

In a medium bowl, whisk the mustard, if using, milk, salt and freshly ground black pepper and cornflour together.

Drain the cooked macaroni and return it to the saucepan. Stir in the milk mixture, bacon, onion and half the grated cheese. Put the saucepan back on the stovetop, and stir over a medium heat for 6–8 minutes until the mixture thickens. Pour into the prepared dish. Sprinkle over the remaining cheese and place under the grill until golden brown, about 5 minutes.

Sprinkle over parsley and chopped tomatoes to serve.

# Garlic Roast Chicken 'n' Vege with Gravy

PREPARATION TIME:
**25 MINUTES**
COOKING TIME: ABOUT
**1 ½ HOURS, PLUS 10 MINUTES**
FOR GRAVY
SERVES **4**

1.5 kg chicken

garlic salt to sprinkle

6 medium potatoes, peeled and halved

4 slices pumpkin, peeled and deseeded

4 small onions, peeled and left whole

4 medium parsnips, peeled and left whole

4 medium carrots, peeled and left whole

5 large kumara, peeled and cut into chunky pieces

3 tablespoons olive oil

**Gravy**

2 tablespoons flour

2 cups chicken stock

salt and freshly ground black pepper to taste

Preheat the oven to 180°C.

Wash the chicken inside and out and pat dry with absorbent kitchen paper. Fold the wings underneath the chicken and tie the legs together with a small piece of string.

Place the chicken in a roasting pan. Sprinkle with garlic salt.

Place the prepared vegetables in a separate roasting pan and drizzle over the olive oil. Stir so that they are well coated, then sprinkle with garlic salt.

Place both pans in the oven and set the timer for 1 ½ hours. Stir the vegetables after 30 minutes and again at 1 hour so that they cook evenly and are coloured golden brown.

To test that the chicken is properly cooked, pierce the thick part of its thigh with a sharp skewer or small knife. If the juice that runs out is clear, then the chicken is cooked. If the juice is still pink, the chicken needs to cook longer (generally, allow 30 minutes per 500 g at 180°C for perfectly cooked chicken). Once it is cooked, remove from the oven. Check the vegetables are nice and crispy but leave them in the oven and turn it off.

Lift the chicken out of the roasting pan onto a serving plate. Cover it with a sheet of aluminium foil and keep it warm in the cooling oven while you make the gravy.

To make the gravy, drain off as much fat as possible from the roasting pan, but retain the juices. Place the pan on the stovetop over a medium heat. Sprinkle in the flour and cook for 1 minute. Use a wire whisk to stir and scrape up any bits of chicken stuck on the pan. Pour in the chicken stock and stir with the whisk. The gravy will thicken and start to boil. If it is too thick, add a little extra water or chicken stock. Season with salt and freshly ground black pepper and pour into a small warmed gravy boat or jug.

Serve the roast chicken and vegetables with the gravy, and a green vegetable like broccoli, peas or green beans.

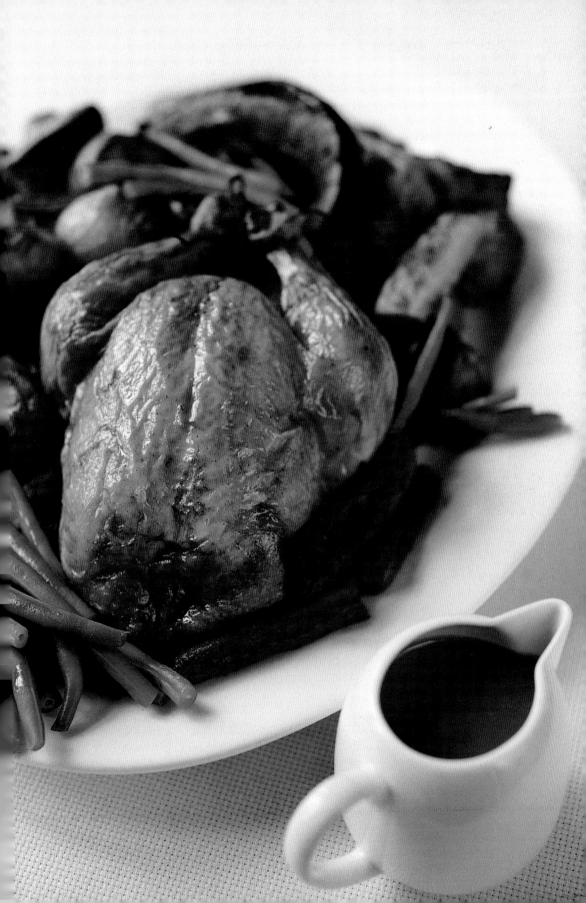

# Glazed Carrots

**PREPARATION TIME:**
**5–6 MINUTES**
**COOKING TIME: 8 MINUTES**
**SERVES 4 AS A SIDE DISH**

4–6 medium-large carrots

2 tablespoons Chelsea Dark Cane Sugar

1 tablespoon margarine or oil

salt and freshly ground black pepper to taste

2 tablespoons chopped parsley (optional)

Scrub and peel the carrots. Slice into discs like 50c pieces.

Place the carrot slices in a saucepan and cover with water. Bring this to the boil and then turn the heat down and simmer for about 5 minutes until the carrots are soft but still quite crisp — not mushy!

Drain the carrots in a sieve or colander. Place the sugar and margarine or oil in the hot saucepan, then put the carrots back in the pot. Toss and season with salt and freshly ground black pepper and mix in the chopped parsley, if using.

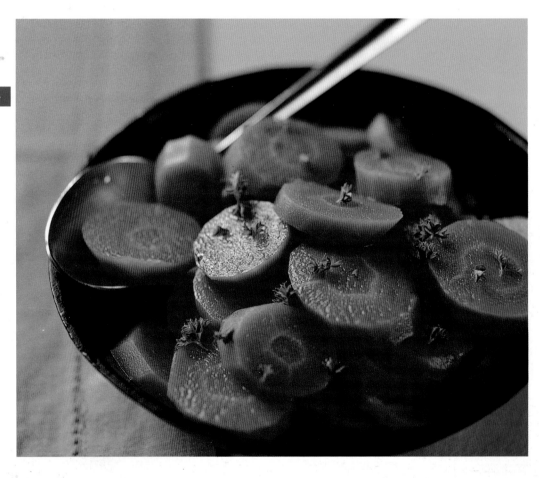

# Cheese Sauce in a Jiffy

Melt the butter or margarine in a small saucepan. Add the flour and stir with a wire whisk for 1 minute. Remove from the heat and whisk in the milk. Return the saucepan to the heat and stir until the sauce thickens.

Season with salt and freshly ground black pepper, then add the grated cheese. Stir until the cheese melts.

**PREPARATION TIME: 2 MINUTES**
**COOKING TIME: 5 MINUTES**
**MAKES 1 CUP**

2 tablespoons soft butter or margarine

2 tablespoons flour

1 cup low-fat milk

salt and freshly ground black pepper to taste

½ cup grated tasty cheese

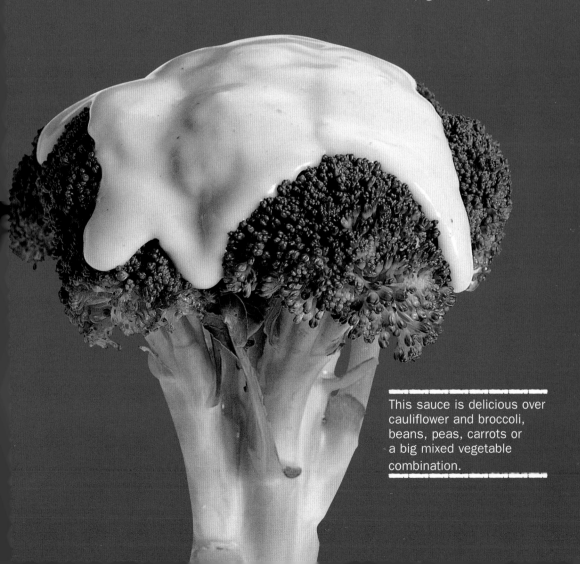

This sauce is delicious over cauliflower and broccoli, beans, peas, carrots or a big mixed vegetable combination.

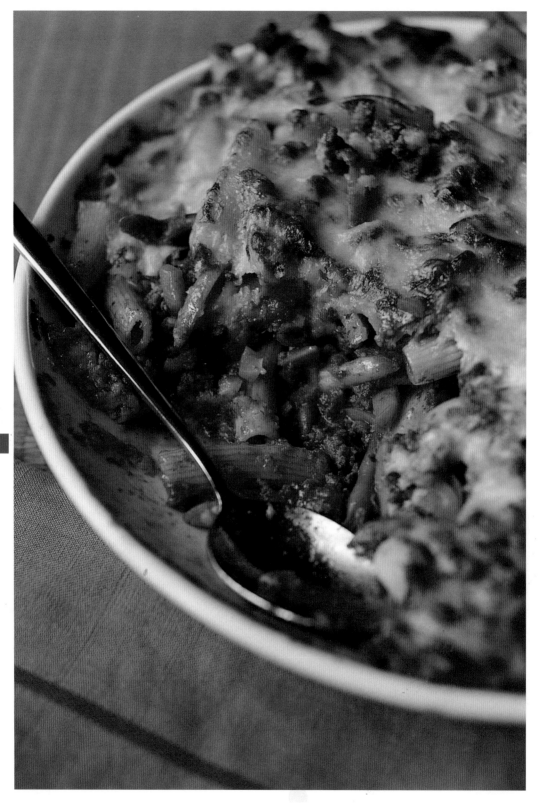

# Hearty Pasta Bake

**PREPARATION TIME:**
**25 MINUTES**
**COOKING TIME: 60 MINUTES**
**SERVES 6**

### Meat sauce

2 tablespoons oil

2 medium onions, peeled and chopped

500 g minced beef or lamb

2 cups spicy pasta sauce from a jar or can

3 tablespoons chopped parsley

salt and freshly ground black pepper to taste

### Pasta

500 g dried penne or rigatoni pasta

4 cups frozen mixed vegetables

### Cheese sauce

100 g butter or margarine

¼ cup flour

3 cups low-fat milk

1 cup grated tasty cheese

3 egg yolks

green salad and bread rolls to serve

Preheat the oven to 180°C. Spray a deep-sided (10 cm deep), 30 cm x 25 cm baking dish or small lasagne dish with non-stick baking spray.

To make the meat sauce, heat the oil in a large frying pan over medium-high heat. Add the onions and cook for 3–4 minutes. Add the mince and cook for 5 minutes, breaking up any lumps. Stir through the pasta sauce and parsley and season with salt and freshly ground black pepper. Let the meat sauce simmer while you cook the pasta.

Cook the pasta in plenty of gently boiling, well-salted water until just tender (al dente), about 10 minutes. Add the frozen vegetables and cook for a further 2 minutes.

Drain in a large sieve or colander. Return to the pot and stir through the meat sauce.

To make the cheese sauce, melt the butter or margarine in a large saucepan. Add the flour and stir with a wire whisk for 1 minute. Whisk in the milk, then the cheese and egg yolks. Stir until the sauce thickens and is smooth.

Pour the meat and vegetable pasta into the prepared dish. Pour over the cheese sauce and bake for about 30 minutes until the top is golden brown.

Serve with a crispy green salad and crusty bread rolls.

**Note:** You can turn the unused egg whites into a Pavlova (see page 96). Egg whites can be stored for up to 3 weeks in a covered container in the refrigerator.

# Lemon Fish & Rice

Rinse the fish fillets in cold water and pat dry with absorbent kitchen paper. Slice the fish into thin strips or fingers, about ½ cm thick.

Heat a large non-stick frying pan. Add the butter and garlic. Heat until the butter is sizzling then add the fish. Stir the fish gently and keep the pan hot and sizzling. Cook for 1 minute only. Add the cooked rice, lemon rind and juice and the parsley. Cook for one more minute just to heat through. Add salt and freshly ground black pepper.

Serve immediately.

**Note:** For 4 cups of cooked rice, bring a saucepan half filled with cold water to the boil, add 1 teaspoon salt and 2 cups rice and boil for 12 minutes, stirring once or twice. Drain in a sieve.

**PREPARATION TIME:**
**15** MINUTES
**COOKING TIME: 3** MINUTES
**SERVES 4**

This mixture is great in pita breads or warm burger buns. You can also add extra vegetables like frozen corn or chopped tomatoes when you add the rice and parsley.

4 medium-sized firm, white fleshed fish fillets, skinned and boned

100 g butter

1–2 cloves garlic, crushed

4 cups cooked rice, well drained (see note)

finely grated rind and juice of 2 lemons

½ cup finely chopped parsley

salt and freshly ground black pepper to taste

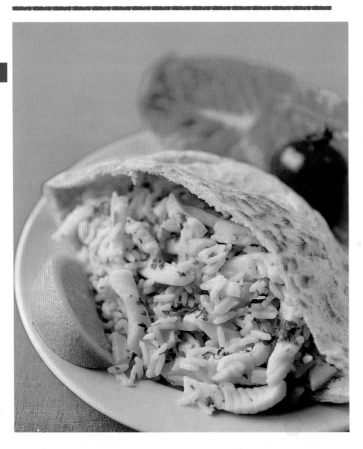

# Noodle Fritters

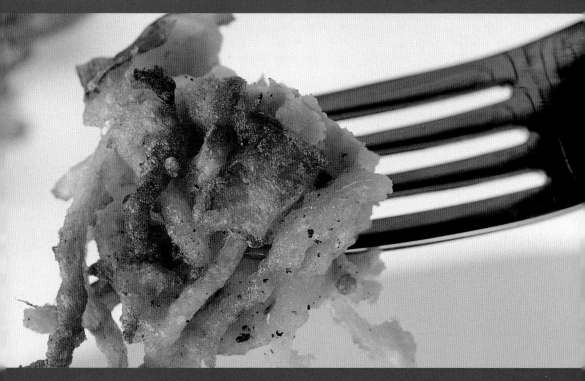

**PREPARATION TIME:**
**10** MINUTES
**COOKING TIME: 15** MINUTES
**MAKES 8 FRITTERS**

2 packets instant noodles, any flavour

1 courgette, grated

2 spring onions, sliced

1 carrot, grated

2 eggs, beaten

2 tablespoons flour

2 tablespoons oil

tomato or soy sauce to serve

Break the noodles up and cook according to the directions on the packet (keep the seasoning mix packets unopened). Drain the noodles and place in a large bowl. Mix in the courgette, spring onions, carrot, eggs, flour and the sachets of seasoning mix.

Heat the oil in a large non-stick frying pan over a medium-high heat.

Ladle in 4 fritters, each one a heaped tablespoon of mixture and fry for 2–3 minutes. Carefully turn over and cook other side. Drain on absorbent kitchen paper while you cook the second batch.

Serve with tomato or soy sauce.

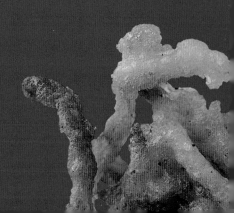

# Sweet 'n' sour Pork Stir-fry

PREPARATION TIME:
**30** MINUTES

COOKING TIME: **15** MINUTES

SERVES **4**

600 g pork schnitzels or lean pork steaks

2 tablespoons oil

3–4 cloves garlic, crushed

1 large onion, peeled and sliced

1 cup pineapple pieces in juice or syrup (1 x 225 g can)

¼ cup tomato or steak sauce

2 tablespoons malt or white vinegar

2 tablespoons Chelsea Soft Brown Sugar

½ red capsicum, deseeded and sliced

½ green capsicum, deseeded and sliced

½ yellow capsicum, deseeded and sliced

1 cup canned baby sweetcorn

1 cup sliced button mushrooms

1 cup fresh or frozen green beans

½ cup bean sprouts

2 tablespoons chopped parsley or coriander

½ cup chicken or beef stock

1 tablespoon cornflour

rice or noodles to serve

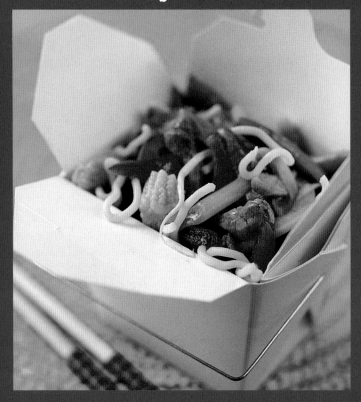

Slice the pork into 5 mm strips or fingers.

Heat the oil in a large non-stick frying pan or wok. Add the garlic and onion and cook for 2 minutes. Add the pork and stir until all the pinkness has gone and it is evenly browned. Add the pineapple pieces (keep the juice aside) and tomato or steak sauce, vinegar, sugar and all the vegetables and parsley or coriander. Stir and cook for 5 minutes.

Mix the stock, cornflour and reserved pineapple juice together and pour into the pork and vegetable mixture. Cook a further 2 minutes until the mixture thickens.

Serve with rice or noodles.

# Fantastic Frittata

**PREPARATION TIME:**
**10** MINUTES
**COOKING TIME: 25** MINUTES
**SERVES 4–6**

2 tablespoons oil

1 medium onion, peeled and chopped

2–3 cloves garlic, crushed

3 large potatoes, peeled and cubed into small dice (1 cm square)

1 cup frozen peas

1 cup sweetcorn (frozen, fresh or canned)

1 carrot, peeled and grated

1 cup small broccoli florets

½ cup chopped parsley

2 cups grated tasty cheese

8 eggs, beaten

salt and freshly ground black pepper to taste

Heat the oil in a large (about 25 cm) non-stick frying pan with an ovenproof handle. Cook the onion and garlic in the pan for 2 minutes. Add the potatoes and cook for 10 minutes, stirring often. Add the other vegetables, parsley and grated cheese. Stir to mix well.

Pour in the beaten eggs and mix through the vegetables. Season with salt and freshly ground black pepper. Turn down the heat and cook for 7–8 minutes. Do not stir.

Meanwhile, preheat the oven grill. Place the frying pan under the grill for 4–5 minutes until the frittata is set and golden brown on top. Leave in the pan for 3–4 minutes before cutting into wedges.

This can be served hot or cold and is great with a salad.

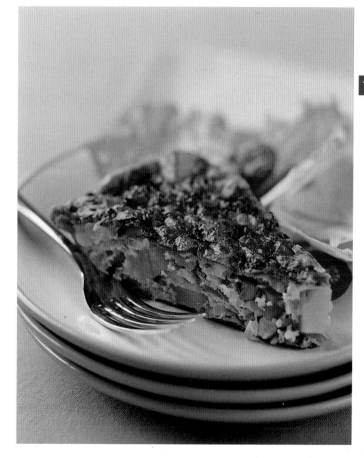

# Desserts

Refresh

Ideas **74**

Scrumptious Ch

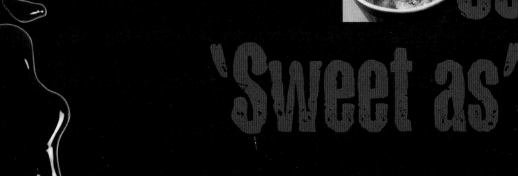

'Quick as'

Soft-freez

Co

'Sweet as'

# Refreshing Funky Fruit Salad Ideas

Fresh fruit salad is one of the best desserts in the world. Simple combinations of prepared fruits in fruit juice or syrup are chilled and served at the end of the meal.

It is nice to have different themes with fruit salad — here are a few good ideas. Keep the fruit salad nice and moist using the natural fruit juices or orange juice, or the juice or syrup from canned fruit.

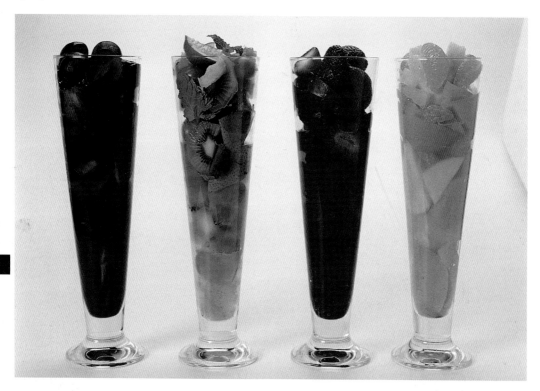

## Black Fruit Salad

purple grapes
dark plums
blackberries
blackcurrants
dark cherries

## Glorious Green Fruit Salad

kiwi fruit
kiwano
green melon
green grapes
green apples
greengage plums
gooseberries

## Racy Red Fruit Salad

strawberries
raspberries
boysenberries
plums
red grapes
cherries
red apples
red pears
watermelon
redcurrants
rhubarb
cranberries

## Go For Gold Fruit Salad

apricots
oranges
mandarins
peaches
nectarines
yellow plums
passionfruit
star fruit
pineapple
banana

# Instant Fruit Sorbet

PREPARATION TIME:
**2** MINUTES, PLUS AT LEAST
**4–6** HOURS FREEZING TIME
COOKING TIME: NO COOKING
REQUIRED
SERVES **2–4**

1 can fruit in syrup:
apricots, peaches,
nectarines, pears, etc
(see note)

Remove the label and lid from an opened can of fruit and freeze it solid. This will take about 4–6 hours, but it is best to leave it overnight.

Run the frozen can under a hot tap to loosen the edges, then tip fruit into the bowl of a food processor. Chop it up a little bit then process the mixture until it is a smooth creamy consistency.

Serve immediately in tall parfait or wine glasses.

**Note:** It is essential that the fruit you use is canned in syrup not fruit juice, as a sorbet needs the sugar in the syrup to work properly.

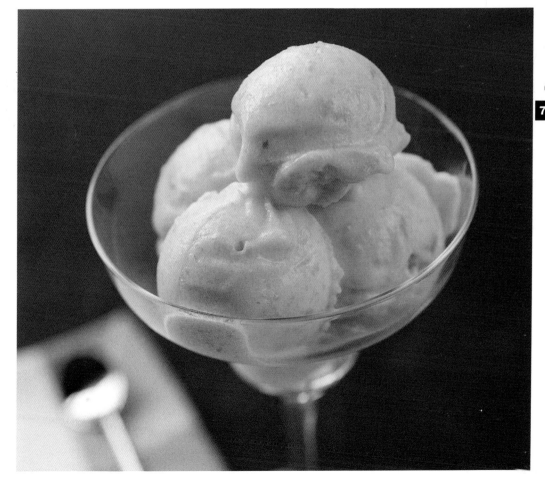

# Scrumptious Choccy Mud Mousse

**PREPARATION TIME:**
**5** MINUTES, PLUS **3** HOURS
CHILLING TIME
**COOKING TIME: 3** MINUTES
**MAKES 6** LARGE OR **10** SMALL
SERVINGS

300 ml cream

250 g dark chocolate chips,
  melts or chocolate bits

3 egg yolks

2 tablespoons Chelsea
  Caster Sugar

whipped cream and
  chopped chocolate or
  pieces of fruit to serve

Pour the cream into a microwave-proof jug or bowl and cook on high for 2–3 minutes until just about to boil, watching carefully so it doesn't overflow.

Place the chocolate, egg yolks and sugar in a blender and pour in the nearly boiling cream. Securely fit on the lid and blend until smooth and well combined. This will take about 30 seconds.

Pour into serving dishes or small glasses. This mousse looks really good in tiny coffee cups or fancy little glasses. Leave to set in the refrigerator for at least 3 hours.

Serve with a dollop of whipped cream and some chopped chocolate or pieces of fruit. Keeps well for 3–4 days in the refrigerator.

## Variations:

- You can substitute white or milk chocolate for the dark chocolate. If using white or milk chocolate, you may find the mixture is sweet enough without adding the caster sugar.
- You can also add flavours such as strawberry or peppermint essence, or the grated rind of an orange.

## Note: You can turn the unused egg whites into a Pavlova (see page 96). Egg whites can be stored for up to 3 weeks in a covered container in the refrigerator.

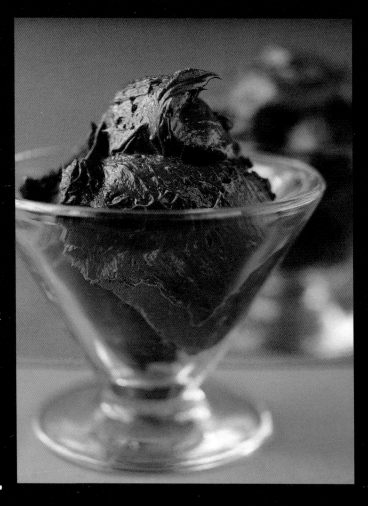

# 'Quick as' Fruit Spongy Puds

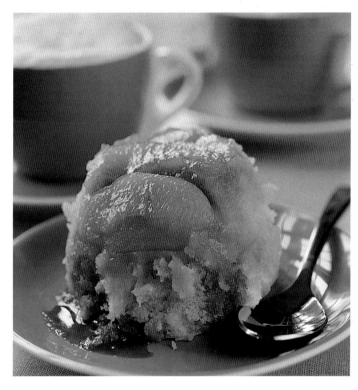

**PREPARATION TIME:**
**10** MINUTES, PLUS
**2–3** MINUTES RESTING TIME
**COOKING TIME: 5** MINUTES
**SERVES 4**

1 cup canned or stewed
   peaches or pears,
   chopped

4 tablespoons jam

50 g butter

1 egg

¼ cup Chelsea Caster or
   White Sugar

1 cup self-raising flour

½ cup low-fat milk

fruit yoghurt, whipped cream
   or ice cream to serve

Spray 4 straight-sided coffee mugs with non-stick baking
spray.

Divide the chopped fruit equally between the mugs.
Spoon a tablespoon of jam over the fruit into each mug.

Place the butter in a medium-sized microwave-proof
bowl. Melt on high power for 30–40 seconds. Beat in the
egg and sugar, then mix in the flour and milk. Spoon the
mixture over the fruit and jam.

Place all four mugs in the microwave and cook together
on high for 3 ½–4 minutes. Rest the puddings for 2–3
minutes in the mugs, then tip out onto individual plates.

Serve with fruit yoghurt, whipped cream or ice cream.

# Soft-freeze Berry Ice Cream

**PREPARATION TIME: 3 MINUTES**
**COOKING TIME: NO COOKING REQUIRED**
**SERVES 4**

3 cups frozen free-flow
   berries: raspberries,
   strawberries, blackberries,
   or a mixture

about ¾ cup Chelsea
   Icing Sugar

1 cup plain or fruit yoghurt,
   or cream or milk, well
   chilled

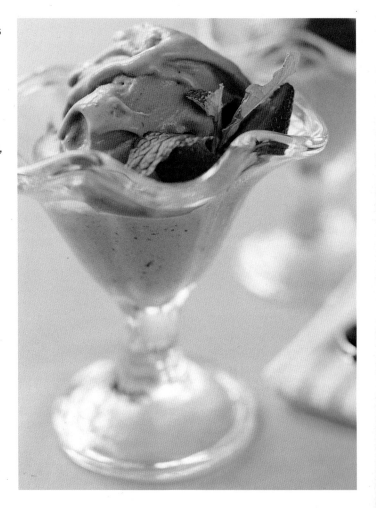

Place the still-frozen berries and icing sugar (you may
need a little more or less depending on the sweetness of
the berries) in a food processor, and process to a frosty
purée. Add the yoghurt, cream or milk and blend to mix
thoroughly.

Serve immediately in tall parfait or wine glasses for a
pretty presentation.

**Note:** This can be refrozen but it never quite reaches
the perfect consistency again, so it is best served
straight away.

# Comfy Apple Crumble

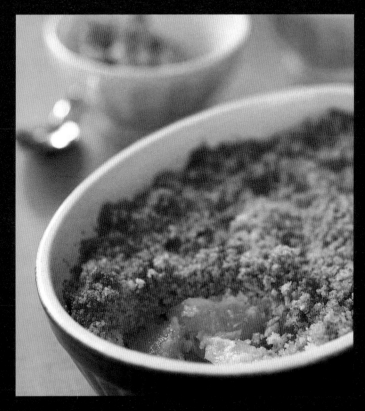

**PREPARATION TIME:**
**15** MINUTES
COOKING TIME: **45** MINUTES
SERVES **4**

6 crisp apples

finely grated rind and juice
of 1 lemon

½ cup apple juice or water

1 teaspoon ground
cinnamon

¾ cup Chelsea Soft Brown
Sugar

¼ cup flour

1 cup rolled oats

100 g butter or margarine

custard, yoghurt, cream or
ice cream to serve

Preheat the oven to 180°C. Spray a pie or lasagne-type dish, about 20 cm x 20 cm, with non-stick baking spray.

Peel, core and slice the apples thinly and spread them in the prepared dish. Mix the lemon juice and apple juice or water together and drizzle over the apple slices.

Place the grated lemon rind, cinnamon, sugar, flour, rolled oats and butter or margarine in a food processor and mix until crumbly. Sprinkle this over the apples.

Bake for 40–45 minutes until bubbly and golden brown.

Serve with custard, yoghurt, cream or ice cream.

## Variations:
Other fruits can be substituted for apples. Try pears, peaches or nectarines, and you can mix together fruits like apples and strawberries or peaches and kiwifruit. Half a cup of raisins or sultanas mixed in with the fruit also adds a nice flavour.

# 'Sweet as' Ice Cream Sauces

## Rich Chocolate Fudge Sauce

PREPARATION TIME: 2 MINUTES
COOKING TIME: ABOUT 10 MINUTES
MAKES: 2 ½ CUPS

1 packet (375 g) dark chocolate melts

300 ml cream

2 tablespoons Chelsea Icing Sugar

Place all the ingredients in a medium saucepan and stir over gentle heat until the chocolate melts. Stir until well combined and smooth.

This sauce will set solid at room temperature, so needs to be served warm.

Store in the refrigerator for up to 10 days.

## Raspberry Sauce

PREPARATION TIME: 2 MINUTES
COOKING TIME: 10 MINUTES
MAKES 1 ½ CUPS

2 cups fresh or frozen raspberries

¼ cup Chelsea Caster Sugar

1 tablespoon cornflour

Mash the raspberries with a fork in a medium-sized saucepan. Stir in the sugar and cornflour and bring to the boil, stirring continuously. Cool.

You can strain out the raspberry pips if you like, but it is fine to leave them in.

Serve warm or cold.

**Note:** For Strawberrry Sauce, use the same measures and methods as the raspberry sauce but replace the raspberries with 2 cups strawberries.

# Caramel Sauce

PREPARATION TIME: **2** MINUTES
COOKING TIME: ABOUT
**6** MINUTES
MAKES **2 ½** CUPS

2 cups Chelsea Soft Brown
Sugar, or try Chelsea Dark
Cane Sugar for a stronger
butterscotch sauce

50 g butter

300 ml cream

1 teaspoon vanilla essence

Combine all the ingredients in a medium-sized saucepan. Stir over a low heat until the sugar has dissolved and the butter has melted. Cool.

Any unused sauce will keep in the refrigerator for up to 10 days.

# Chocolate Sauce

PREPARATION TIME: **2** MINUTES
COOKING TIME: **10** MINUTES
MAKES **1 ½** CUPS

2 tablespoons cornflour

¼ cup cocoa

2 tablespoons cold water

1 cup hot water

¼ cup Chelsea Caster Sugar

25 g butter

1 teaspoon vanilla essence

In a small saucepan, blend the cornflour and cocoa with the cold water to make a smooth paste. Stir in the hot water, sugar and butter. Stir over a medium heat until the mixture boils and thickens, about 8 minutes. Stir in the vanilla.

Cool and store in the refrigerator. The sauce may need warming before use if it becomes too hard in the refrigerator.

# Bacon-wrapped Water Chestnuts

**PREPARATION TIME:**
**15** MINUTES
**COOKING TIME: 15** MINUTES
**MAKES ABOUT 36**

1 can whole water
chestnuts

12 rashers rindless streaky
bacon

garlic salt to sprinkle

36 bamboo skewers,
medium length

Preheat the oven to 200°C.

Drain the water chestnuts — there should be 33–36 in the can. Cut each bacon rasher into three and wrap one piece around a water chestnut. Carefully skewer on the end of a bamboo skewer and lay in a shallow roasting dish. Sprinkle with garlic salt.

Bake for about 15 minutes until the bacon is crispy.

Serve warm. These can be reheated in the oven or microwave.

## Variations: Try a pitted prune wrapped in bacon. These don't need any garlic salt.

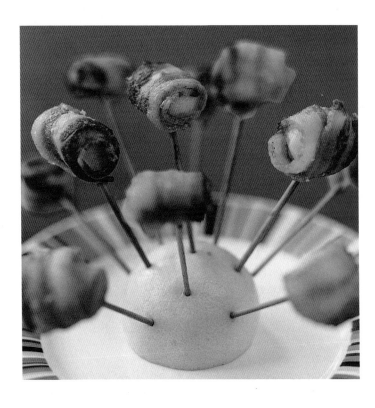

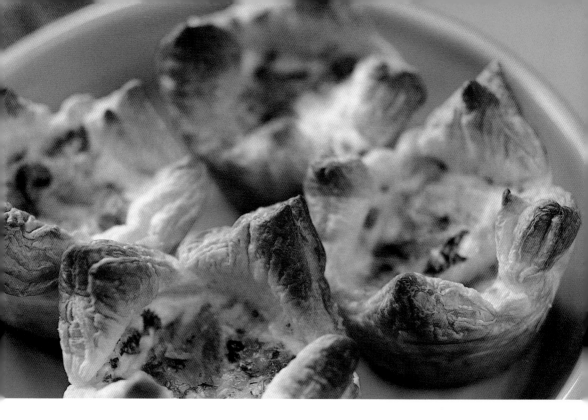

# Individual Bacon & Egg Pies

Preheat the oven to 200°C. Spray three mini muffin trays with non-stick baking spray.

Using a 4–5 cm round cookie cutter, press out 36 circles of pastry. Press the pastry into the sprayed muffin cups. Divide the bacon, cheese and peas between the pies.

Beat the cream or milk, eggs, parsley, salt and pepper together until well mixed. Using a small jug pour this mixture into each pie, filling them halfway up.

Bake for about 20 minutes until puffed up and golden with the pastry crispy and browned. Cool in the tins for about 10 minutes until you can easily handle them without oven gloves. Carefully twist and lift each little pie out of the muffin tins.

These can be eaten warm or cold. They are great for lunch boxes or picnics and make a lovely finger-food for parties.

**PREPARATION TIME: 30 MINUTES**
**COOKING TIME: 20 MINUTES**
**MAKES 36 MINI PIES**

3 sheets frozen flaky or puff pastry, thawed

6 rashers lean rindless bacon, cut into small pieces

2 cups grated tasty cheese

1 cup frozen peas

1 cup cream or milk

4 eggs

2 tablespoons chopped parsley

½ teaspoon salt

½ teaspoon pepper

# Fudgilicious Brownies

**PREPARATION TIME:**
**10** MINUTES
**COOKING TIME: 35** MINUTES
**MAKES ABOUT 15** BIG FUDGEY PIECES

375 g dark chocolate, or
    1 packet dark chocolate
    melts

200 g butter

2 cups Chelsea White Sugar

3 eggs

1 teaspoon vanilla essence

1 cup flour

1 cup mixed nuts (cashews,
    walnuts, pecans, peanuts,
    etc), chopped

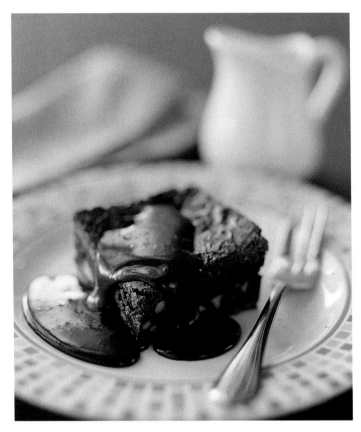

## Jo's Tip:

THIS MAKES A FABULOUS BASE FOR A DESSERT. JUST ADD A SCOOP OF ICE CREAM AND CHOCOLATE FUDGE SAUCE (SEE PAGE 80). GARNISH WITH STRAWBERRIES OR RASPBERRIES. BROWNIES CAN ALSO BE FROSTED WITH CHOCOLATE ICING (SEE PAGE 30) OR DUSTED WITH SIFTED CHELSEA ICING SUGAR.

Preheat the oven to 180°C. Line a medium-sized sponge roll tin, about 18 cm x 25 cm, with non-stick baking paper.

In a large microwave-proof bowl melt the chocolate and butter together on high power for 3–5 minutes, then stir until smooth and well blended. Mix in the sugar, eggs and vanilla, then stir in the flour and nuts. Pour into the prepared tin.

Bake for 30–35 minutes or until a skewer inserted into the centre comes out with fudgey crumbs. The brownie should be quite fudgey and sticky, not dry and cake-like.

Cool in the tin and cut into bars. Store in an airtight container.

# Guacamole

PREPARATION TIME: **5** MINUTES
COOKING TIME: NO COOKING
REQUIRED
MAKES **1** CUP

1 ripe avocado

2 teaspoons lemon juice

½ cup low-fat sour cream

2 tablespoons chopped
parsley

salt and freshly ground
black pepper to taste

1 teaspoon sweet chilli
sauce (optional)

corn chips, Crostini or Pita
Crisps to serve

# Pita Crisps

PREPARATION TIME: **5** MINUTES
COOKING TIME:
**10–15** MINUTES
MAKES A BIG PILE, ABOUT **80**
PIECES

5 pita breads, plain,
wholemeal or garlic
flavoured

¼ cup olive oil to brush, or
olive oil spray

about 1 ½ teaspoons garlic
salt to sprinkle

Cut the avocado in half, remove the stone and scoop out the flesh into a bowl. Mash with a fork. Mix in the lemon juice, sour cream and parsley. Season with salt and freshly ground black pepper and sweet chilli sauce, if using.

Serve with corn chips, Crostini (see page 89) or Pita Crisps (see below).

Best eaten within 24 hours, store in the fridge, covered tightly with plastic wrap.

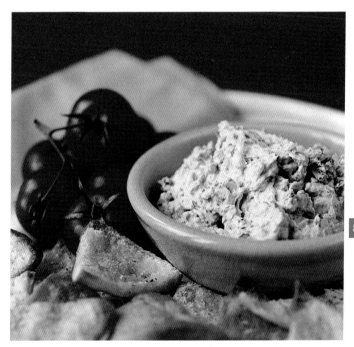

Preheat the oven to 200°C.

Using scissors, cut the pita breads in half, then quarters, then eighths. Peel the bread open making two wedges from each piece. Using a pastry brush or sprayer, coat the rough sides of the pita bread with olive oil and place them, oiled side up, in a large roasting dish. Sprinkle with garlic salt.

Bake for 10–15 minutes until golden and crisp.

Cool on a wire cake rack and store in an airtight container.

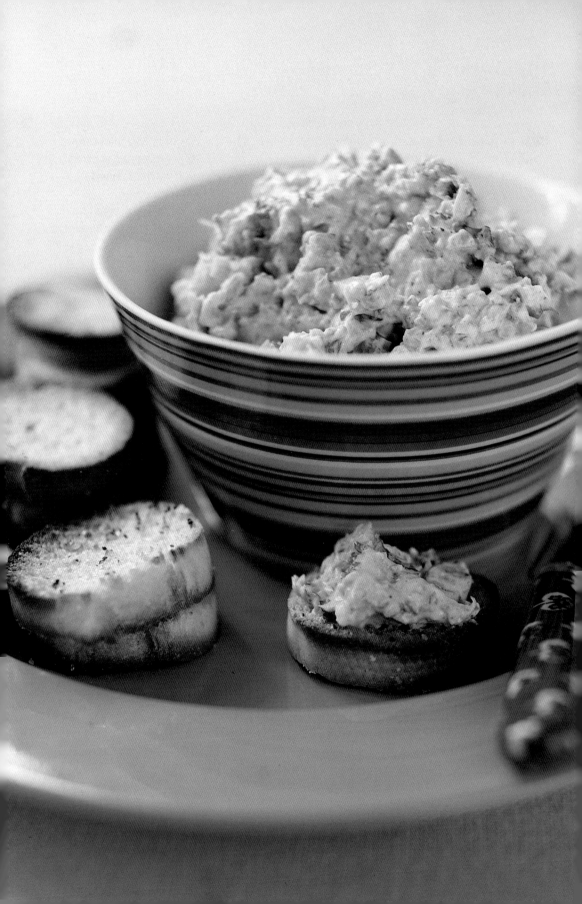

# Chickpea & Yoghurt Dip

**PREPARATION TIME: 5 MINUTES**
**COOKING TIME: NO COOKING REQUIRED**
**MAKES 2 CUPS (ENOUGH FOR 4–6 PEOPLE)**

1 cup canned chickpeas, drained

2 cups natural unsweetened yoghurt

½ cup chopped parsley

salt and freshly ground black pepper to taste

1 teaspoon sweet chilli sauce or to taste

½ teaspoon mild curry powder

corn chips, Crostini or Pita Crisps to serve

Place all ingredients in a food processor and mix until well combined and smooth.

Serve in a small bowl with corn chips, Crostini (see below) or Pita Crisps (see page 87).

# Crostini

**PREPARATION TIME: 10 MINUTES**
**COOKING TIME: 10–15 MINUTES**
**MAKES 36–40**

1 loaf of French bread (baguette)

¼ cup olive oil to brush, or olive oil spray

about 1–1 ½ teaspoons garlic salt to sprinkle

Preheat the oven to 200°C.

Cut the bread into 1-cm thick slices. Using a pastry brush or sprayer, coat both sides of each slice of bread with olive oil, then lay flat on two baking trays or roasting dishes. Sprinkle with garlic salt and bake for 10–15 minutes until golden brown and crisp.

Cool on a wire cake rack and store in an airtight container.

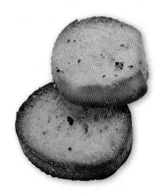

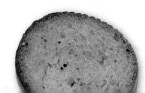

# Iced Chocolate Cupcakes

Preheat the oven to 180°C. Place paper cupcake cases in a set of 12 muffin trays.

Place the flour, cocoa and sugar in a large bowl. Place the butter in a measuring cup and add the eggs, then fill up to the 1 cup measurement with milk. Beat this into the dry ingredients until smooth.

Fill cupcake cases three-quarters full. Bake for 15 minutes.

To serve, either dust the cupcakes with icing sugar, or ice with Chocolate Icing (see page 30).

(see page 30)

**PREPARATION TIME:**
**5** MINUTES, PLUS **5** MINUTES FOR THE ICING
**COOKING TIME: 15** MINUTES
**MAKES 12**

1 cup self-raising flour

2 tablespoons cocoa

¾ cup sugar

50 g butter, melted

2 eggs

about ¾ cup low-fat milk

Chelsea Icing Sugar to dust (optional)

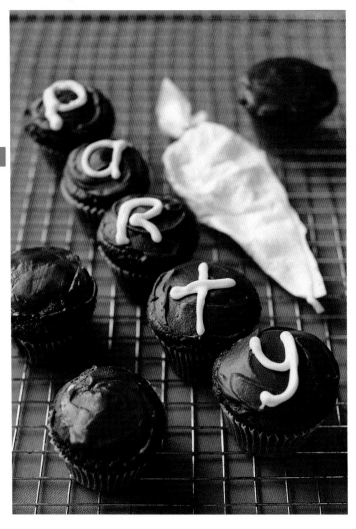

## Jo's Tip:

MELT **10–15** WHITE CHOCOLATE MELT BUTTONS IN A SMALL ZIPLOCK PLASTIC BAG IN BURSTS OF **30** SECONDS ON MEDIUM (OR HALF POWER) IN THE MICROWAVE.
AFTER EACH **30** SECONDS, SQUISH THE BAG TO MIX THE CHOCOLATE ABOUT UNTIL IT IS MELTED AND SMOOTH. WITH SCISSORS, SNIP THE CORNER OFF THE BAG AND USE TO PIPE OUT NAMES OR **HAPPY BIRTHDAY** — ONE LETTER PER CUPCAKE. WHOOPS! THAT'S **13** LETTERS — YOU'LL NEED TO MAKE **2** BATCHES TO WRITE YOUR NAME AS WELL!

# Best Birthday Bash Choccy Cake

**PREPARATION TIME:**
**15** MINUTES
**COOKING TIME: 35** MINUTES
**MAKES A LARGE CAKE THAT**
**CAN BE CUT INTO 16 PIECES**

2 cups Chelsea Caster
   Sugar

3 cups self-raising flour

2 teaspoons baking soda

½ cup cocoa

4 eggs, separated

2 cups low-fat milk

2 tablespoons malt vinegar

2 tablespoons Chelsea
   Golden Syrup

2 teaspoons vanilla
   essence

1 ½ cups oil (canola, soya
   or light olive oil)

**Filling**

150 ml cream, whipped

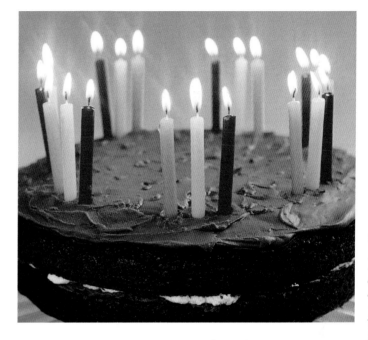

Preheat the oven to 180°C. Spray two 23–25 cm cake tins (preferably spring-sided tins) with non-stick baking spray, and line the bases with non-stick baking paper.

Set out 3 medium-large bowls.

Into the first bowl place the sugar, flour, baking soda and cocoa. Mix well.

Into the second bowl place the 4 egg yolks, milk, vinegar, golden syrup, vanilla and oil. Mix well.

Into the third bowl place the egg whites. Beat these with a hand-held electric mixer until soft and frothy white.

Pour the liquid ingredients from the second bowl onto the dry ingredients in the first bowl, and mix well together. A hand-held electric mixer will really combine the ingredients well. Gently fold in the beaten egg whites with a spoon, until just combined. Pour the mixture into the two prepared tins and bake for 35 minutes.

Cool in the tins for 5 minutes, then tip out and cool completely on a wire cake rack. Peel off the paper.

To serve, spread one cake with the whipped cream and place the other one on top. Ice the top (and sides if you desire) with Chocolate Icing (see page 30) and don't forget the birthday candles!

# Simple Sushi

**PREPARATION TIME:**
**20–30** MINUTES
**COOKING TIME: 35** MINUTES
**MAKES 20–30** PIECES

2 ½ cups sushi or short-grain rice

4 cups cold water

2 teaspoons salt

100 ml rice wine vinegar

1 tablespoon Chelsea Caster Sugar

5 nori seaweed sheets

wasabi paste to taste (a traditional very hot Japanese horseradish paste)

5 slices smoked salmon

about 100 g pickled ginger

1 firm but ripe avocado, peeled, stoned and sliced

5–10 chives

soy sauce, extra wasabi and pickled ginger to serve

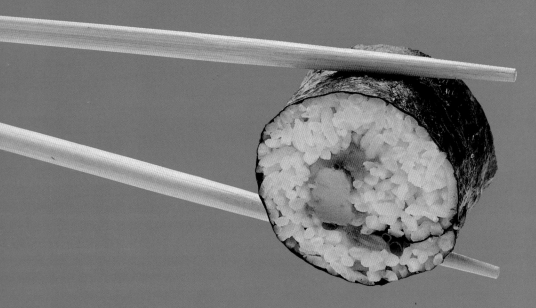

**1** Wash the rice in a sieve under cold running water for 2 minutes. Drain. Place rice and cold water in a medium saucepan. Bring to the boil and gently boil for 8 minutes. Turn off the heat, cover the saucepan with a lid and let it rest for 25 minutes to completely absorb the water. Fluff the rice with a fork and mix in the salt, vinegar and sugar. Cool to room temperature.

**2** Place a sheet of nori, shiny side down, on a bamboo sushi mat or a sheet of baking paper. Working with wet hands, spread a fifth of the rice in an even layer on the nori, leaving a 3 cm strip of nori on one edge uncovered. Spread a very thin smear of wasabi paste on the rice at the edge closest to you (be careful as this can be fiery hot!). Now lay lines of smoked salmon, pickled ginger, avocado slices and chives next to the wasabi.

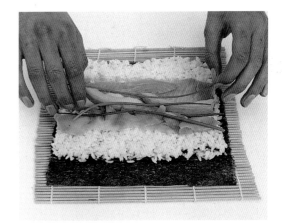

**3** Using the bamboo mat or baking paper to help you, roll up the sushi as firmly as possible. Start at the edge closest to you. Using a pastry brush, dampen the uncovered nori with a little water to help seal the join.

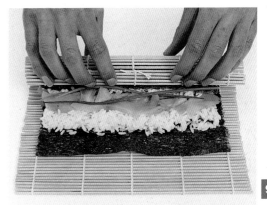

**4** Using a very sharp knife, dipped in water after each slice, cut the sushi rolls into bite-sized pieces.

Serve the sushi within an hour or store covered in the refrigerator. Serve with a tiny dish of soy sauce, wasabi and extra pickled ginger.

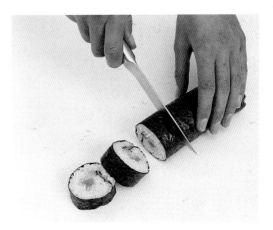

**Note:** If you find rolling the sushi too difficult, you can sandwich up the layers with rice, nori and filling and cut up like a little club sandwich.

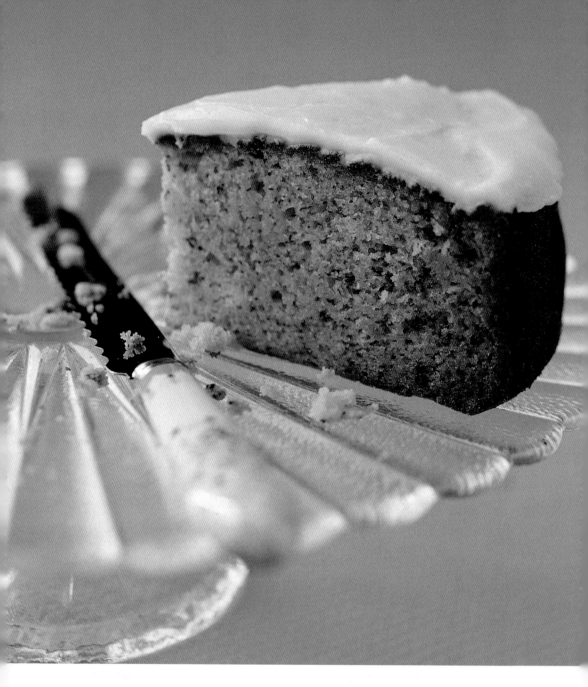

# Cream Cheese Frosting

**PREPARATION TIME: 5 MINUTES**
**COOKING TIME: NO COOKING REQUIRED**
**MAKES 1 CUP**

100 g cream cheese, softened

2 cups Chelsea Icing Sugar

finely grated rind and juice of 1 lemon

Beat all ingredients together until well mixed, fluffy and smooth. Spread over the cooled cake.

# Brill Banana Cake

**PREPARATION TIME:**
**20 MINUTES**
**COOKING TIME: 50 MINUTES**
**MAKES A 20 CM CAKE, BIG**
**ENOUGH FOR 8 GOOD SLICES**

1 cup Chelsea White Sugar

100 g butter, melted

3 eggs

3 bananas, mashed

½ cup low-fat milk

1 teaspoon baking soda

150 ml plain or fruit yoghurt
 (apricot is very nice)

2 cups flour

3 teaspoons baking powder

Preheat the oven to 160°C. Spray a 20–22 cm round springform baking tin with non-stick baking spray. Line the base with baking paper.

Beat the sugar, butter and eggs until thick and creamy. Add the mashed bananas and beat well.

Heat the milk in a small microwave-proof bowl or a glass jug in the microwave until nearly boiling (about 1 minute).

Stir the baking soda into the milk and then stir this into the banana mixture. Add the yoghurt, flour and baking powder. Mix well and pour into the prepared cake tin.

Bake for 45–50 minutes until the cake is cooked in the middle and just pulling away from the edges of the tin. Cool in the tin for 5 minutes then release the spring sides and cool completely on a wire cake rack.

When completely cold, ice with either Lemon Icing or Cream Cheese Frosting.

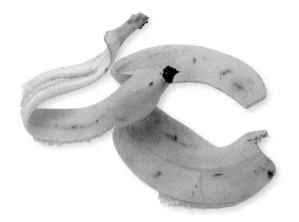

# Lemon Icing

**PREPARATION TIME: 5 MINUTES**
**COOKING TIME: NO COOKING**
**REQUIRED**
**MAKES ½ CUP**

25 g butter or margarine

finely grated rind and juice
 of 1 lemon (strain the
 juice to remove the pips)

2 cups Chelsea Icing Sugar

Place the butter, lemon rind and juice in a small microwave-proof jug or bowl. Microwave on high for 30–40 seconds until the butter is melted. Beat in the icing sugar to make a fluffy icing. Spread over the cooled cake.

# Pavlova

**PREPARATION TIME:**
**15** MINUTES
**COOKING TIME: 1 ½ HOURS**
**SERVES 4–6**

3 egg whites, at room
temperature

1 cup Chelsea Caster Sugar

1 teaspoon vanilla essence

1 teaspoon malt or white
vinegar

2 teaspoons cornflour

whipped cream or yoghurt
and fresh fruit to serve

Preheat the oven to 120°C. Line a baking tray with baking
paper.

Place the egg whites into a large metal, china or glass
bowl (not plastic as the egg whites won't beat up as well).
Beat until thick and stiff. A hand-held electric mixer is
ideal for this job. Gradually, just 1 teaspoon at a time, add
the sugar, beating in well after each teaspoon is added.
The mixture slowly gets glossy, thick and shiny. Don't
rush adding the sugar, as this part of pavlova making is
very important. The whole sugar-adding process should
take about 8–10 minutes. Beat in the vanilla, vinegar and
cornflour.

Spoon the mixture onto the prepared tray and spread
out in a circle the size of a small plate (about 18 cm
diameter). Bake for 1 ½ hours until the pavlova is crisp
and dry and easily lifts off the paper. Don't be tempted to
turn up the heat as you want a nice dry, pale pav, not a
brown burnt one.

Cool completely on a wire cake rack before covering
with cream or yoghurt and sliced fresh fruit.

96

## Variations:

● To make a special rolled pavlova, preheat the oven
to 180°C. Follow the same instructions but spread the
mixture out into a rectangle shape, about 18 cm x 25 cm.
Bake at the higher temperature for 20 minutes. Remove
from the oven and cool completely. Spread with cream
or yoghurt and fruit, then roll up into a log starting from
the long side. Don't worry that the pav crumbles and
cracks — this looks fine. Place on a serving dish and dust
generously with icing sugar.

● This recipe can also be used for meringues. Simply
follow the same instructions up to spreading out on the
tray. For meringues, spoon out 10–25 small blobs of
mixture with plenty of space in between them. Bake at
120°C for approximately 30–35 minutes until crisp and
dry and you can lift them easily from the paper.

**Note:** This recipe easily
doubles to make a big
party-sized pavlova to feed
8–12 people.

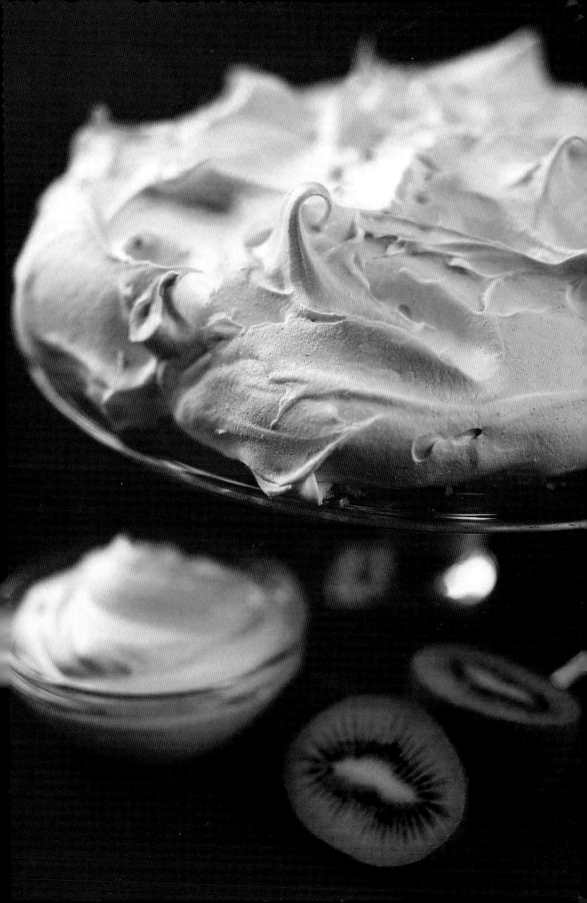

# Fundraising

Slice 100   Coc...

Truffle Treats 102   G...

Royal Icing 104   Lus...

Sherbet Lollyp...

Bubbles 108

Chocolate Fudgecake

ut Ice **101** Chocolate

gerbread People **104**

ous Lemon Honey **106**

os **107** Peanut Butter

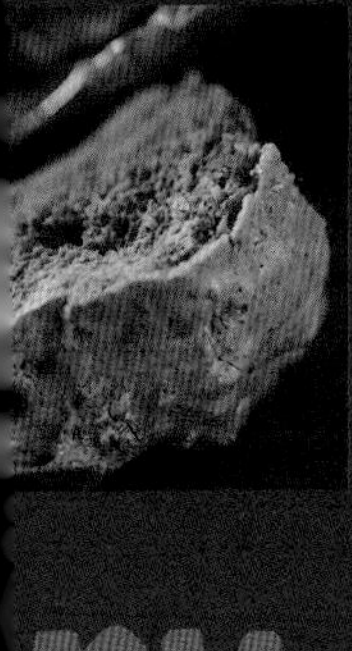

Hokey Pokey **108**

ry Vanilla Fudge **109**

# Chocolate Fudgecake Slice

1 packet (225 g) digestive
   or wine biscuits

125 g butter

½ cup Chelsea White Sugar

1 egg, lightly beaten with a
   fork

2 tablespoons cocoa

2 teaspoons mixed spice

1 cup chopped nuts
   (walnuts, peanuts, etc)

1 cup sultanas

1 teaspoon vanilla essence

Line a 20 cm x 20 cm square cake tin with baking paper.

Crush the biscuits in a food processor, or place them in a large heavyweight plastic bag, seal and crush with a rolling pin.

Melt the butter in a large microwave-proof bowl on high for 30–45 seconds. Stir in the sugar and egg. Microwave for 30 seconds, then continue to cook in bursts of 30 seconds, stirring in between, until the mixture starts to boil. Stir in the cocoa, mixed spice, nuts, sultanas, vanilla and biscuit crumbs. Press into the prepared tin and chill.

When chilled, ice with Chocolate Icing (see page 30). Allow the icing to set, then cut into squares or bars.

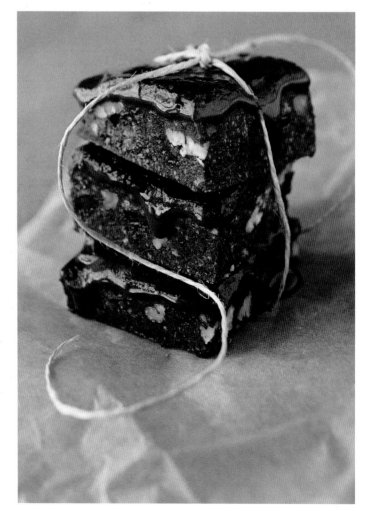

# Coconut Ice

**PREPARATION TIME: 5 MINUTES**
**COOKING TIME:**
**25–30 MINUTES**
**MAKES 25–30 PIECES**

100 g butter

1 cup low-fat milk

6 cups Chelsea Icing Sugar

1 teaspoon salt

1 cup desiccated coconut

2 teaspoons coconut
  essence

## Jo's Tip:

**FOR PINK COCONUT ICE
ADD A DROP OF RED FOOD
COLOURING WITH THE
COCONUT. FOR THE
TRADITIONAL TWO-TONE
EFFECT, MAKE A BATCH OF
WHITE, THEN A BATCH OF
PINK, POURING THE PINK ON
TOP OF THE WHITE AFTER
BEATING THEN LEAVE IN THE
TIN TO COOL AND SET.**

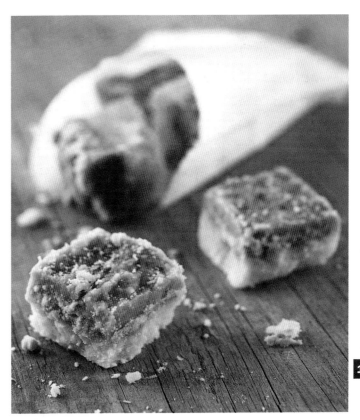

Fundraising

Spray a 20 cm x 20 cm cake tin with non-stick baking spray.

Place the butter, milk, icing sugar and salt in a medium-sized saucepan and heat gently until the sugar dissolves. Bring the mixture to the boil and keep the heat sufficient to just maintain the boil, stirring only occasionally, until the mixture reaches soft-ball stage (120°C). To test without a thermometer, fill a glass with cold water. Now drop a little of the mixture into the water. The mixture is ready when the drips form soft little balls in the cold water. Add the coconut and coconut essence and remove from the heat. Cool for 5–10 minutes, then beat until the mixture thickens.

Pour into the prepared tin. Allow to cool and cut into squares.

# Chocolate Truffle Treats

**PREPARATION TIME:
30 MINUTES, PLUS 3–4
HOURS CHILLING TIME
COOKING TIME: NO COOKING
REQUIRED
MAKES 60 TRUFFLES**

125 g butter or margarine

1 can (400 g) sweetened
condensed milk

1 cup Chelsea Icing Sugar

2 cups crushed digestive or
wine biscuit crumbs

¼ cup cocoa

2 teaspoons mixed spice

1 cup raisins, sultanas or
chopped pitted prunes

375 g dark or milk
chocolate melts to dip
truffles

**1** Cover a baking tray with
aluminium foil.
  Melt the butter or
margarine in a large
microwave-proof bowl
on high power. Stir in
the condensed milk and
microwave on high for
1 minute. Stir in the icing
sugar, biscuit crumbs,
cocoa, mixed spice and
dried fruit. Mix well to
combine.

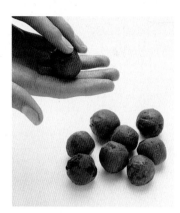

**2** Roll teaspoonfuls
of the mixture into large
marble-sized balls and
place on the prepared tray.
Place in the refrigerator to
chill until hard. This should
take about 3–4 hours in the
refrigerator or 1 hour in the
freezer.
  Place the chocolate
melts in a microwave-proof
jug or small bowl. Cook
on medium power in 30
second bursts, stirring
after each burst until the
chocolate is just melted
and runny. There are good
instructions for melting on
the side of the packets of
melts.

**3** Dip one cold truffle
at a time into the melted
chocolate.

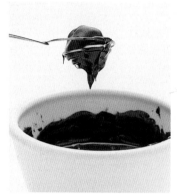

**4** Swirl it around to
coat well and lift carefully
out onto the aluminium foil-
lined tray to set. A special
dipping fork makes the job
very easy or use 2 bamboo
skewers or chopsticks.

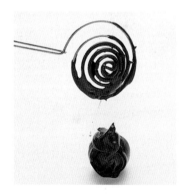

## Jo's Tip:

**INSTEAD OF DIPPING IN
MELTED CHOCOLATE, AFTER
ROLLING OUT YOUR BALLS,
DIP IN CHOCOLATE HAIL OR
COCONUT, THEN CHILL.**

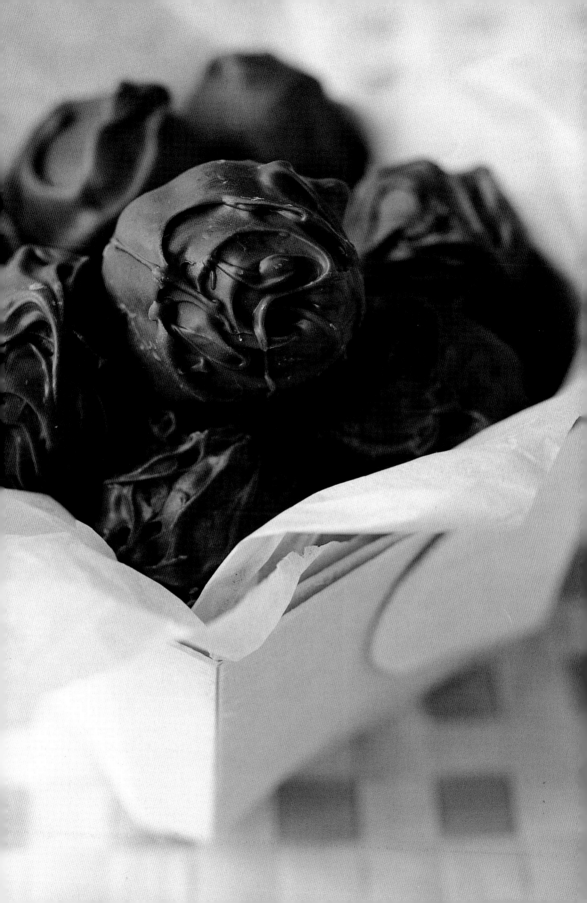

# Gingerbread People

PREPARATION TIME:
20 MINUTES, PLUS 3 HOURS
CHILLING, PLUS 5 MINUTES FOR
THE ICING
COOKING TIME: 15 MINUTES
MAKES 40

125 g butter

1 cup Chelsea Dark Cane Sugar

2 teaspoons baking soda

1 teaspoon salt

2 teaspoons ground ginger

1 teaspoon mixed spice

1 teaspoon ground cinnamon

1 cup Chelsea Treacle

½ cup warm water

7 cups flour

In a large bowl, beat the butter and sugar until creamy. Mix in the baking soda, salt, ginger, mixed spice and cinnamon. Mix in the treacle and warm water then slowly mix in the flour. Add a little extra flour if the mixture is too moist to roll out. Cover with plastic wrap and chill in the refrigerator for at least 3 hours. The mixture can be stored in the refrigerator for up to 5 days.

Preheat the oven to 180°C. Cover two baking trays with baking paper or spray with non-stick baking spray.

Divide the dough into 4. Taking one of these quarters at a time, roll out to 1 cm thick on a floured bench or board. Cut out gingerbread people, or other shapes, using a cookie cutter. Use a wide spatula to transfer to the prepared trays. Bake for 12–15 minutes until firm and dark brown. Cool for 2 minutes on the tray then remove to cool completely on a wire cake rack.

When cold, ice with Royal Icing, using a piping bag to outline details such as eyes, mouth, buttons, etc.

# Royal Icing

PREPARATION TIME: 10 MINUTES
COOKING TIME: NO COOKING REQUIRED
MAKES 1 ½ CUPS — ENOUGH FOR 40 GINGERBREAD PEOPLE

2 egg whites

2 tablespoons cold water

1 tablespoon strained lemon juice (no pips or fibre)

2 ½ cups Chelsea Icing Sugar

Place all the ingredients in a large bowl and beat with a hand-held electric mixer until fluffy, thick and shiny. Spoon into a piping bag or you can use a small ziplock plastic bag with a small hole cut out of the corner. Pipe on faces and clothing details.

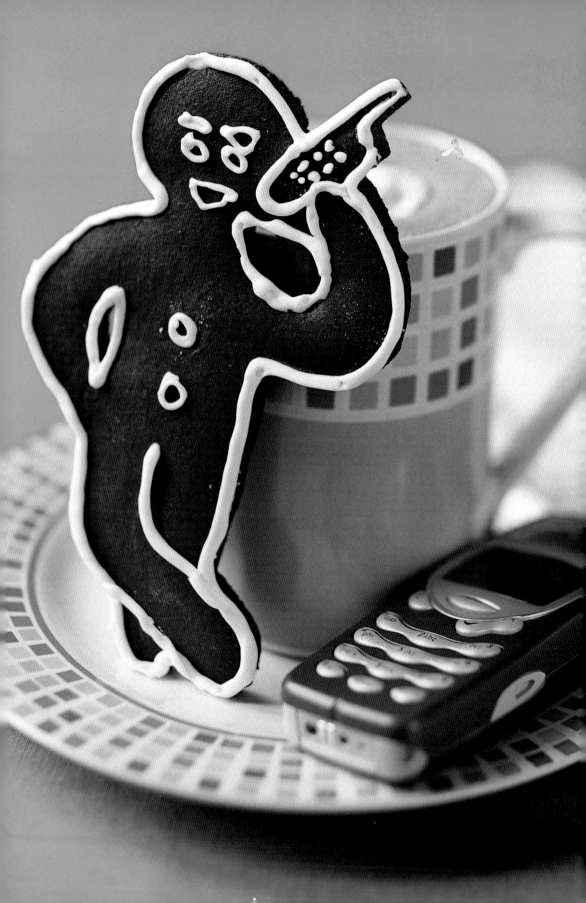

# Luscious Lemon Honey

**PREPARATION TIME:**
**10** MINUTES
**COOKING TIME: 8–10** MINUTES
**MAKES 2** CUPS

4 eggs

1 ½ cups Chelsea White Sugar

100 g butter, cut into little pieces

finely grated rind and juice of 2 lemons

Place the eggs and sugar in a large microwave-proof bowl or jug. Whisk with a wire whisk until well combined. Add the butter, lemon rind and juice. Cook on high for 8–10 minutes, stirring every minute until the mixture is smooth, thick and creamy. Cool for 5 minutes then pour into warm clean jars. Seal when cold and store in the refrigerator.

Perfect on toast, ice cream or serve with lemon cakes or in tarts.

## Jo's Tip:

TO MAKE PASSIONFRUIT HONEY, REPLACE THE LEMON MEASURE ABOVE WITH ¼ CUP PASSIONFRUIT PULP AND THE GRATED RIND AND JUICE OF 1 LEMON. FOLLOW THE SAME INSTRUCTIONS.

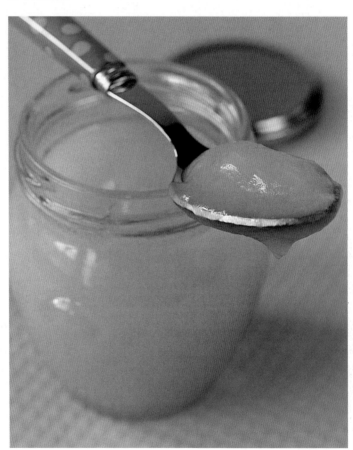

# Sherbet Lollypops

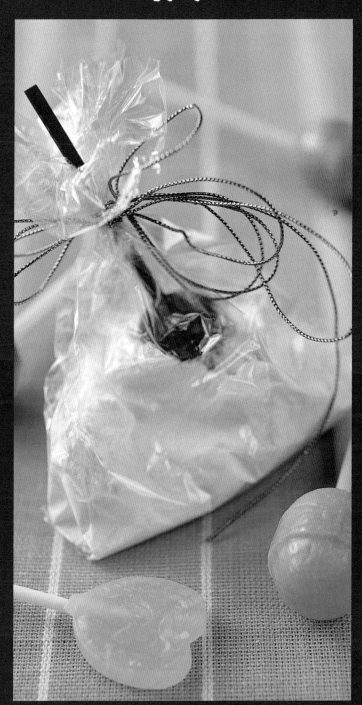

**PREPARATION TIME: 5 MINUTES**
**COOKING TIME: NO COOKING REQUIRED**
**SERVES 6**

1 cup Chelsea Icing Sugar

2 tablespoons of powdered drink crystals (Refresh, Raro, etc)

1 ½ teaspoons citric acid

1 ½ teaspoons tartaric acid

1 teaspoon baking soda

6 lollypops

Put all the ingredients, except the lollypops, into a bowl and mix thoroughly. Spoon into little cellophane bags, then insert a lollypop in each bag and seal securely.

To eat, lick the lollypop and dip it into the sherbet.

# Peanut Butter Bubbles

**PREPARATION TIME: 5 MINUTES**
**COOKING TIME: 4 MINUTES**
**MAKES 36–40**

1 cup crunchy peanut butter

125 g butter or margarine

2 cups rice bubbles

2 cups Chelsea Icing Sugar

Place the peanut butter and butter in a large microwave-proof bowl. Microwave on high for 30 seconds. Stir, then cook on high for another 45 seconds–1 minute until the butter is melted. Stir in the rice bubbles and icing sugar. Roll into balls the size of large marbles and place on a tray or large plate in the refrigerator to set and chill.

Store in a covered container in the refrigerator.

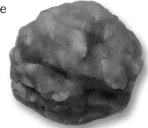

# Hokey Pokey

**PREPARATION TIME: 2 MINUTES**
**COOKING TIME: 5 MINUTES**
**MAKES 15–20 CHUNKS**

5 tablespoons Chelsea
   White Sugar

2 tablespoons Chelsea
   Golden Syrup

1 teaspoon baking soda

Spray a 20 cm x 20 cm cake tin with non-stick baking spray.

Place the sugar and golden syrup in a saucepan. Heat gently, stirring constantly, until the sugar has dissolved. Increase the heat and bring to the boil. Boil for 2 minutes. Stir occasionally if necessary to prevent burning and sticking to the bottom. Remove from the heat and add the baking soda. Stir quickly as the mixture froths up rapidly!

Pour immediately into the prepared tin. Leave until cold and hard, then break into pieces.

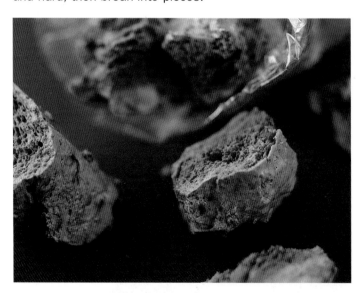

# Very Vanilla Fudge (in the Microwave)

**PREPARATION TIME: 3 MINUTES**
**COOKING TIME: 10–15 MINUTES**
**MAKES ABOUT 36 PIECES**

100 g butter

1 cup Chelsea White Sugar

1 can (400 g) sweetened condensed milk

4 tablespoons Chelsea Golden Syrup

2 teaspoons vanilla essence

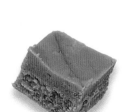

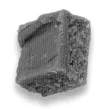

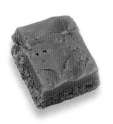

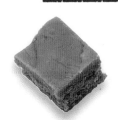

Spray a 20 cm square cake tin with non-stick baking spray.

You will need to use a large microwave-proof measuring jug or pyrex bowl — make sure it can be used at high temperatures (an ordinary plastic bowl will melt when you make fudge).

Place all the ingredients, except the vanilla, in the bowl and microwave on high power for 1 minute. Stir, then cook a further 2 minutes, then stir again. Repeat this for a total of 10 minutes. (If you have a sugar thermometer it should read 120°C.) To test without a thermometer, fill a glass with cold water. Now drop a little of the mixture into the water. The mixture is ready when the drips form soft little balls in the cold water. You may need to cook another 2–4 minutes to achieve this stage.

Remove carefully from the microwave and place the bowl on a wooden board to protect the bench. Add the vanilla — be careful as it can splatter and create steam. Beat the fudge for 4 minutes with a wooden spoon or you can use a hand-held electric mixer. The mixture loses its shine and starts to become very thick and set.

Quickly pour into the prepared tin. When cool, mark into squares, then allow to set and cool completely in the tin.

Fundraising

---

## Variations:

● For a nutty version, add ½ cup chopped mixed nuts just before you pour into the tin
● Raisin Fudge, add ½ cup raisins just before you pour into the tin
● Chocolate, add 3 tablespoons cocoa to the sugar mixture before cooking
● Coconut, add 3 tablespoons desiccated coconut with the vanilla
● Strawberry, add 2 teaspoons strawberry essence instead of the vanilla

---

# Glossary

**Bake:** To cook with hot, dry air. This is done in the oven.

**Baking Powder & Baking Soda:** Rising agents used to make dough rise during baking. Can be acid, like cream of tartar, or alkali, like bicarbonate of soda. Baking soda makes the dioxide gas bubbles that make Hokey Pokey bubble up.

**Baste:** Spoon or brush the juices and marinade over meat or poultry during roasting to keep it moist.

**Batch:** A quantity of food made at one time, such as a batch of biscuits or cookies.

**Batter:** An uncooked mixture that is thin enough to pour, usually has egg, flour and a liquid, like pancake batter.

**Beat:** Mix ingredients together by stirring vigorously, usually with a wire whisk or electric mixer.

**Blanch:** Briefly put food into boiling water without cooking it — used to remove skins from tomatoes.

**Blend:** Mix ingredients thoroughly, or mix ingredients in an electric blender.

**Boil:** Heat a liquid until bubbles keep rising and breaking on the surface.

**Chill:** Put in the refrigerator until cold.

**Chop:** Cut food into small, uneven pieces. Coarsely chopped is big pieces, finely chopped is small pieces.

**Combine:** Mix ingredients together.

**Cream:** Beat together butter and sugar until the mixture is pale and fluffy and looks a bit like whipped cream.

**Dice:** Cut into small cubes.

**Dough:** An uncooked mixture soft enough to be worked with the hands but too stiff to pour, like bread dough.

**Drain:** Pour off liquid, generally by putting it through a strainer or colander.

**Dust:** To cover very lightly with a flour or icing sugar. Icing sugar is often sprinkled or dusted over cakes or muffins before serving.

**Fry:** Cook food in hot fat or oil.

**Garnish:** Decoration, not necessarily edible, added to the finished dish to make it look nice. Parsley is the most common garnish.

**Grate:** Rub against a grater to shred into small pieces.

**Grease:** Rub the surface of a tray or cake tin with butter or oil to stop the mixture from sticking during cooking.

**Knead:** Work dough with the heel of your hand.

**Marinate:** Soak meat or poultry in a mixture of oil, vinegar, citrus juice or wine and flavourings to make it tender and add flavour.

**Melt:** Heat a solid, such as butter, until it becomes liquid.

**Pinch:** The amount of dry ingredient that you can pick up between your thumb and forefinger.

**Poach:** Cook food gently in liquid at the simmer point, so that the surface of the liquid is just below boiling point.

**Preheat:** Heat the oven up before putting the food in. It usually takes about 15 minutes for an oven to come up to baking temperature.

**Roast:** To cook in the oven, usually used for meat or vegetables.

**Sift:** Shake dry ingredients through a sieve to get a soft, airy texture and remove any lumps or impurities.

**Stir-fry:** Quick method of frying in a little oil. The food must be cut into small pieces and moved around until cooked. Usually done in a wok over a high heat.

**Zest:** The brightly coloured outer layer of peel of a citrus fruit such as an orange or lemon.

# Index